SECOND EDITION

UP

Taking Ophthalmic Administrators and Their Management Teams to the Next Level of Skill, Performance, and Career Satisfaction

SECOND EDITION

UP

Taking Ophthalmic Administrators and Their Management Teams to the Next Level of Skill, Performance, and Career Satisfaction

Corinne Z. Wohl, MHSA, COE

John B. Pinto

CRC Press
Taylor & Francis Group
Boca Raton London New York

CRC Press is an imprint of the
Taylor & Francis Group, an **informa** business

First published 2021 by SLACK Incorporated

Published 2024 by CRC Press
2385 NW Executive Center Drive, Suite 320, Boca Raton FL 33431

and by CRC Press
4 Park Square, Milton Park, Abingdon, Oxon, OX14 4RN

CRC Press is an imprint of Taylor & Francis Group, LLC

Cover Artist: Lori Shields

ISBN: 9781630919207 (pbk)
ISBN: 9781003526858 (ebk)

DOI: 10.1201/9781003526858

Dedication

This book is dedicated to:

Our mothers, Alice and Irene, among whose many wisdoms were the value of hard work, the importance of proper English, and the fact that girls and boys are equal (way before that was a popular opinion).

Our fathers, Richard and Julian, each 49% wise and 51% wise-guys. You both chose free-spirited, brave, and unconventional paths, emboldening us to do the same.

Our kid siblings, Matt and Laura, who as professional educators (golf and sociology) keep teaching us how similar these two disciplines are to the business of ophthalmology … and that love, patience, and humor improve it all.

Our children, Rachael and Graham, who miraculously inherited our best bits and skirted the disaster of all our worst habits. How did you turn out to be so perfect?

Our champions, with special mentions to Paula, Steve, Sherri, Big Al, both darling Trevors, and an inspirational spa day from the amazing Victoria Eye Team.

And each other, as life partners, business partners, and shipmates on this grand voyage.

Contents

About the Authors

Corinne Wohl, MHSA, COE is a practice management consultant, executive coach and president of C. Wohl & Associates, Inc. She earned her Master's of Health Services Administration degree at The George Washington University in Washington, DC, and has 35 years of hospital administration, physician practice management, and health care consulting experience.

Corinne's passion is to work in a trusting relationship with surgeons and administrators to help advance their life's work and achieve their personal best. She is best known for bringing her detailed business and clinic operations experience to bear on practices of all sizes, while simultaneously helping clients see the longer term, big picture of where they are taking their enterprises.

Corinne specializes in ophthalmic leadership effectiveness, practice operations enhancement, financial benchmarking and analysis, management team development, and executive coaching for managers and physician leaders. She enjoys working with a diverse range of clients, from solo practitioners to large institutions.

A featured keynote speaker and program facilitator during her long career in eye care, Corinne is a frequent contributor to *Ophthalmology Management*, *Ocular Surgery News*, *EyeWorld*, *Administrative Eyecare*, and *Cataract & Refractive Surgery Today*. She has been an active member of the American Society of Ophthalmic Administrators, including serving as *Administrative Eyecare* magazine's editorial board chair and as a member of the National Board for the Certification of Ophthalmic Executives. She holds a certificate from the Yale School of Management.

John B. Pinto is the most-published author in America on ophthalmology practice management topics. He founded J. Pinto & Associates, Inc, in 1979. Since then, he has provided strategic planning, operations, and marketing advice to pharmaceutical companies, basic science centers, hospitals, multispecialty clinics, and single-specialty facilities.

For 40 years, a majority of the firm's work has served ophthalmic practices ranging from small solo practices to high-volume market leaders, teaching centers, and ophthalmic product companies. He has been active as a practice consultant in North America and Europe and has worked and lectured in South America and Asia.

John is best known as a strategic planning and economic advisor to practices large and small. In addition to covering most dimensions of modern practice operations management, he is a career advisor, providing individual coaching and contract negotiation services to new graduates and midcareer employed ophthalmologists. His professional life today is rounded out with succession planning, practice valuations, partner dispute mediation, merger/acquisition counsel, and leadership development for administrators and physicians.

A prolific writer, Pinto is the author of several books beyond the text you now hold:

- *John Pinto's Little Green Book of Ophthalmology, Sixth Edition*
- *Simple: The Inner Game of Ophthalmic Practice Success, Second Edition*
- *Ophthalmic Leadership: A Practical Guide for Physicians, Administrators, and Teams, Second Edition*
- *Turnaround: Twenty-One Weeks to Ophthalmic Practice Survival and Permanent Improvement*
- *Ten Eyecare Practices: Benchmarks for Success*
- *Cash Flow: The Practical Art of Earning More From Your Ophthalmology Practice*, written with Anne Rose
- *The Efficient Ophthalmologist*
- *Legal Issues in Ophthalmology: A Review for Surgeons and Administrators*, written with Alan Reider and Allison Shuren
- *The Women of Ophthalmology*, written with Elizabeth Davis, MD
- *Marketing Your Ophthalmic Practice*

John is a member of the editorial boards of *Ocular Surgery News*, *Ophthalmology Management*, and *Premier Surgeon*, and a regular contributor to other eye care publications.

• • •

Corinne Wohl and John Pinto practice together in San Diego, California, and are available for individual, practice-wide, and institutional consulting to supplement this book. Please contact them at:

Corinne Wohl, MHSA, COE
C. Wohl & Associates, Inc
(609) 410-2932
czwohl@gmail.com
www.wohlconsulting.com

John B. Pinto
J. Pinto & Associates, Inc
(619) 223-2233
pintoinc@aol.com
www.pintoinc.com

FOREWORD

Imagine a perfectly terrific, highly competent, and confident practice administrator from the 1980s traveling forward in a time machine a couple of decades to run an ophthalmic practice. "What's this MIPS, and what about MACRA, ACO, HIPAA, and EHR? Have I joined the Army?! What's this half-million-dollar laser? Have I joined a hospital?! What's this jumble of baffling accountant-speak from private equity firms? Have I joined an investment bank?!"

Our time traveler would certainly find it hard to orient in the world we know as contemporary ophthalmic practice management. And so, too, do most of us, even though we've had years and years to accommodate to a changing, complexifying, multiplexing career.

As hard as it is for administrators to keep up, consider the colleagues above us, the doctors we serve, and the colleagues we directly supervise, our beleaguered department heads. As practice leaders, we need to not only keep up with blistering change but soothe frazzled nerves up and down the ranks.

This new book by Corinne Wohl (who in recent years left practice administration to consult around the world) and her partner, well-known consultant and author, John Pinto, fills a longstanding hole in our business library.

As you are about to read, *UP* works at several levels. As a primer for newer managers, as a tactical guide for experienced managers, and as a bank of exercises and worksheets you can directly apply at all levels of your organization. I believe that this book will become a classic that is especially valuable to our mid-level managers and those seeking to enhance their management knowledge and professional growth.

In the eye care industry, most middle managers are former high performers in billing, or in the technical department, or at the front desk. They excelled in their line role, so we moved them up to management. They are good learners, they come to work on time, they stay away from negative behaviors, and they are truly a pleasure to have on your team.

But these qualities alone are not enough.

More often than not, while their hearts and heads are in the right place, our up-through-the-ranks managers fail more often than we would like to admit. This happens primarily because they have never been trained to manage. They have been given the keys to your veritable Ferrari of a practice, but no behind-the-wheel instruction. And worse, no owner's manual in the glove compartment. This new book is a start in the right direction.

UP will provide you with tools you need to keep your ophthalmology practice running at peak performance. By laying out for you both basic and advanced dimensions of administration and mid-level management, Corinne and John will help you select better management candidates, assist your star performers, and proceed with the painful staff pruning work that every administrator must undertake. Some of this new text is in workbook format, which makes it easy for you to move beyond theory and dive right in with specific actions and exercises.

With 75 combined years of work in hospital, private practice, and corporate settings, Corinne and John have a wealth of resources to share with you in this new book. Corinne has become the go-to executive coach for new ophthalmic administrators in this country and a source of seasoned counsel for some of the most senior executives in our field.

Please enjoy *UP* as I have. As a practical guide, a source of inspiration on the toughest days, and as a reminder of the direction that we all want to be heading.

—*Suzanne D. Bruno, MBA*
Margate, New Jersey

Suzanne D. Bruno, MBA is a Past President of the American Society of Ophthalmic Administrators and contributor to *Administrative Eyecare*. She is the administrator of Horizon Eye Care, a regional eye care practice in southern New Jersey with 10 physicians and more than 80 staff members.

Introduction

The idea for this book emerged chiefly from Corinne's executive coaching work with some of the smartest, hardest-working administrators and managers in the business. We hope this book will make it easier for you to discover what you know, what you don't know, what you need to know, and how to bridge that gap.

The field of ophthalmic practice management has undergone sweeping changes in the last 35 years. Practice management has professionalized at a faster pace in eye care than in other medical specialties for a number of reasons:

- Higher staff-to-provider ratio, generating more human resources challenges
- Diverse service and payer base: primary to tertiary care, cosmetic care, retail
- Higher economic production per provider obliges financial skills not present in lower-yielding specialties
- Because we operate largely in a geriatric sector, even low-ambition practices must deal with high growth and fast-paced organizational change because of the rapid growth in demand from the "Age Wave" rolling over the United States

A common thread linking all of these challenges is that success in the average practice rests on a cohort of just a few mid-level department managers reporting to an administrator. When this business team is skilled, aligned, and well led, the practice thrives. And vice versa.

While ophthalmologists spend more than a decade in formal training, and rank and file staff can master their finite tasks in a year or two, mid-level managers and their supervising administrators must hold the entire team together in an environment demanding very high and very broad skills, with disproportionately little formal education in most cases ... and all in a setting where continuous personal career development is often underresourced.

Although the average eye surgeon works in only a couple of private practices in the course of a 30+ year career, and the average ophthalmic practice administrator or mid-level manager works in fewer than five eye care practices in the course of a career, their experiences are very different. Ophthalmologists may see thousands of patients over the years, but they have a chance to solve the same presenting conditions over and over again, which results in a level of mastery not witnessed in many professions. By contrast, practice managers solve a diversity of different "presenting conditions" ... they are more like family doctors than ophthalmic subspecialists. Mastery is harder to achieve.

At the same time, administrators and mid-level managers get to go deep and understand their organization's detailed operations when they stay in one position for many years. But this can be a little like a doctor just working with the same few patients over and over again. Lots of depth, but very little breadth.

By contrast, consultants may not go very deep (we're told that often!), but what we lack in depth we gain in breadth. In a single year we, the authors, work with scores of organizations. Together, we have more than 75 years of combined heath care business experience. As you'll read in these pages, we think that doctors and administrators and managers and consultants working together is the best approach, delivering the best health care for patients, the best careers for health care executives, and the best financial performance for practice owners.

Collectively, having worked with thousands of practice managers around the world, we have had the privilege to view ophthalmic practice management from all angles. Large and small practices. Thriving practices and failing ones. Harmonious practices and practices where the doctor-owners are at war with each other or competitors in their markets.

We have developed this workbook to fill in the gap between the deeper textbooks we have published over the years and the intense immersion training that occurs at national conferences.

UP is a powerful, step-wise workbook designed to meet administrators and department managers wherever they happen to be in their careers. We hope it helps to take you tangibly to the next level.

This workbook addresses the chief skills needed to be a manager today, breaking each of them down into digestible learning units. We believe that administrators will find this new workbook useful to coach and develop their management teams. It is also meant as a supplemental source for physician-leaders, who can only accomplish their board-level goals through a well-oiled management staff.

Why do some managers succeed and others fail? What makes some administrators superior? We hope that *UP* will answer these questions for you and provide the support you need to move to your next level of performance and career satisfaction.

—Corinne Wohl, MHSA, COE
—John B. Pinto
San Diego, California

Section I

Core Administrator Skills

CHAPTER 1

Essential Administrator Skills

Good, better, best. Never let it rest.
'Til your good is better and your better is best.
—St. Jerome

You got to be rigorous in your appraisal system.
The biggest cowards are managers who don't let people know where they stand.
—Jack Welch

The good you do today will often be forgotten.
Do good anyway.
—Mother Teresa

How good are you? Where do you stand? Formally and regularly evaluating your skills as an administrator will enhance your career and your practice at the same time. Yet it is surprisingly common for practices not to provide a formal performance appraisal on senior management staff, until problems arise, so many administrators are obliged to assess their own performance. And even if the doctors in your practice are good at giving feedback, you will be a better professional if you adopt the habit of regular self-assessment. Successful practice management encompasses hundreds of tasks that need to be performed well. If even some of these tasks fall short, the practice feels stressed, misguided. The numbers will show it. And the practice board will know it.

Wohl C, Pinto JB. *UP: Taking Ophthalmic Administrators and Their Management Teams to the Next Level of Skill, Performance, and Career Satisfaction, Second Edition* (pp 3-11).

Success-bound administrators are hungry to know how they can improve their skills and how they can help make owners happier and the practices at large more successful.

Highly skilled administrators make the job look easy. In high-functioning settings, we hear employees say, "I'm not exactly sure what our administrator does, but this place *really* runs well."

Just as a missed step in cataract surgery can result in disaster, a single management misstep, can lead to a poorly run practice. It is easy to overlook what skills should be present, especially if you have been working in the same practice for a long time.

Unless you are vigilant with your personal education, the skills you arrived with long ago may have softened or become obsolete. You may be trying to catch up. You *should always* be trying to catch up or, better yet, stay ahead! A formal inventory and evaluation of these skills can keep you sharp and leaning into your current position … or prepare you for your next professional posting.

• • •

The best administrators in the most successful practices understand the strategic details and management nuances required to wrangle a large group of people of various ages, intellects, career goals, and commitment down the same path at the same time.

But no great administrator we have ever met—and we've worked with the best—excels in every category. The wisest managers are uncomfortably aware of their weakest areas … *and then work on these areas.*

An evaluation of your performance as an administrator needs to start with written expectations and goals that you, the practice owners, and managing partner agree on. An updated position description is a good place to begin. By adding specific and measurable goals to this base document, you are at the same time creating a specific checklist for your own career success. Revisit this list on a quarterly basis together with your practice's managing partner, communicating about the progress and any barriers to achievement that may have occurred. Annually, hold a formal meeting with the board where you are prepared to discuss achievements, failures, and new goals.

• • •

It's an important observation that the best administrators are not the ones who are running around merely looking busy. When you were very young, perhaps someone read the story to you of the Tortoise and the Hare from *Aesop's Fables:* "The Tortoise plodded on and plodded on, and when the Hare awoke from his nap, he saw the Tortoise just near the winning-post and could not run up in time to save the race."

Although you work in eye care, and you probably think that what one *SEES* is pretty important, appearances can be deceiving when gauging your own output and efficiency and that of your staff. For example, the most laconic-appearing practice managers—those who seem to dawdle through their week—may be the ones getting the most accomplished for their practice. The first time we understood this was not watching an ophthalmic manager, but watching a carpenter, who was working on a Texas client's private residence.

Mike was the slowest-moving tradesman we had ever seen. And yet, not a single motion was wasted. Nine hours a day, Mike moved deliberately from task to task. The result—working almost entirely by himself to build a 6,000-square-foot house in under a year—was a masterpiece created in less time, and at less cost, than could be accomplished by the typical five-person crew.

Here's what we saw:

Mike would walk from his truck when he arrived on the job site, past the building materials staged out front. As he walked past a stack of wooden studs, he would grab an armload and move to the closest place they were needed (where he also had a saw plugged in and ready to go). With a fluid series of motions—but by no means quickly—he would measure, cut, and hammer in place one stud after the other. Observed for just a few minutes, Mike looked like a very slow worker, indeed. But Mike's slow pace camouflaged the fact that he never *stopped* working. He was in constant, purposeful action for the entire day.

Seeing Mike in slow-steady action, compared to other carpenters, brought to mind some of the most effective administrators and office managers we've worked with through the years. These executives are not so much the caffeinated Hare-paced set, but the ambling Tortoise, plowing ahead without wasted motion and little drama.

As a practice administrator, here are eight things you can do to relax, know that the job is getting done, and bring more efficiency to the process of running your enterprise.

1. **Judge your performance by outcomes, not just time and motion.** Yes, showing up is important. But a punctual administrator rolling out 30% profit margins isn't doing the practice any favors. Quite often, the manager who stays on hours after the practice has closed, or who has to take home mounds of unfinished work each night, is not so much dedicated as drowning and inefficient.
2. **Make sure major time is spent on major tasks.** To stretch the construction analogy, a building's foundation, walls, and roof should get most of the attention ... arranging the landscaping so it's just right is way, way down the list. You should apply most of your time to buttressing the core assets of the organization: the doctors, the staff, the facility, and the sources of new patients.
3. **Avidly delegate to help ensure a calm environment.** The Hare-like administrator, hopping around in anxious circles with hair on fire, is a sure sign of underdelegation. If you are presently underdelegating, it's unlikely you will change your habits much just by reading these words. It will help to walk through the following five-step exercise:
   a. List, in the greatest possible detail, all of your management job functions (this is going to be a long list, potentially 100 items or more).
   b. Next to each item, write a number between 1 and 10, with "1" being of little importance to the organization, and "10" being of very high importance.
   c. Then, go back to each item and score it on the same 1 to 10 scale, but this time with "1" being very easy to delegate to someone else (inside or outside the practice) and "10" being essentially impossible to delegate.
   d. Multiply the two scores and rank order all of the resulting composite scores.
   e. Commit to delegating everything below a selected composite score.

Here's an example, looking at four job functions:

Job Function	Importance to the Practice *1 = Low importance* *10 = High importance*	Ease of Delegation *1 = Easy to delegate* *10 = Impossible to delegate*	Composite Score
Preparing for board meetings	9	9	81
Screening new hires	8	7	56
Biweekly payroll	7	2	14
Stocking exam rooms	5	1	5

In this example, the first two job functions are very important, and difficult to delegate, and they have high composite scores. They definitely should be retained by the administrator. The last two job functions are less important, easier to delegate, and should probably be passed on to others.

4. **Be clear about communicating deadline expectations.** If you work with a Tortoise mid-level manager who is eventually going to get things done quite well—but who, along the way, will generate in you a high level of anxiety about, "How are we coming along with Project X?"—then make sure you've worked out a regular time for your manager to report in to you. And, by all means, tell your manager, "When I don't hear from you about Project X, I assume it's not getting done, which makes me uncomfortable, so please keep me in the loop."
5. **Make sure your mid-level managers are clear about the outcomes you seek.** We've talked to department managers who thought the goal was cutting costs at every turn and then heard their administrator say, "We're not that interested in cost-cutting. We want to grow the practice at the fastest possible pace and understand that this may require extra outlays and some waste." Ideally, you, your board, and your management teams have co-developed a written plan for the next 3 to 5 years (5 to 10 years for larger institutions), with sequential, measurable hallmarks. (It's like Mike the carpenter having written blueprints for the house he was building.)
6. **Do one thing at a time.** Okay, maybe two things. Excessive multitasking leaves lots of unfinished balls up in the air to fall on your head. The most effective ophthalmic executives will delve into one or two projects at a time, resolving each issue intelligently, deeply, and finitely, so that it doesn't arise again. Less effective managers can have dozens of projects in the works (and appear to be highly accomplished) but only have time to apply temporary, incomplete solutions. This results in the same issues arising repeatedly, and never really achieving closure.

7. **The basics are essential.** Communication should be clear, and with increasing practice scale, formal and written. Meetings should be effective, with frequency proportional to practice scale (larger practices need *far* more meetings than small practices). Financial and volumetric benchmarking data have to be timely, and equally well understood by both lay managers and physician-owners. A means of tracking forward progress with projects is essential. (As a practice, you keep dated chart notes on each patient; your managers should have an analogous, transparent system in place so that you and your board know where each project stands.)
8. **Appearances count.** Readers above a certain age may remember Deputy Barney Fife (played on TV by Don Knotts), the overly excitable sidekick to the town sheriff, played by Andy Griffith. At the first sniff of petty crime, Barney (the Hare) would be dashing all over the little town of Mayberry, begging to put his one allotted bullet to work. Andy (the Tortoise) always sorted things out calmly by the end of the episode. The self-collected, effective administrator listens calmly as a provider downloads the "emergency" of the hour, settling an overwrought surgeon's nerves and assuring with a tone of confidence that all will be well. Less effective managers will send their excitable, thoroughbred doctor into even higher orbit, validating the provider's anxiety, while dropping everything else to investigate.

• • •

What follows is a simple consulting tool we've used for years to help administrators raise their consciousness, celebrate their strengths and pry into their weakest areas. Applied with a healthy dose of honesty, this self-test can point the way to real improvements.

Administrator's Scorecard

The following is a list of 10 important attributes possessed by some of the best administrators. This list is by no means complete, and no administrator could be expected to have top scores on all of these attributes. Circle the most appropriate number for each item and add up the total. The maximum score is 20 points.

Score each item on this 10-item list based on the following scale:

2 = This attribute is present in abundance.

1 = This attribute is present but not yet fully developed.

0 = This attribute is absent.

#1. Raw Career Tenure in Health Care Services Management/Leadership

It takes about 25,000 hours of hard work and a very heavy tuition bill to turn a bright high school graduate into a rookie eye surgeon. In another 10,000 hours or so beyond this you have a 35-year-old ophthalmologist who most readers would be comfortable having operate on a distant and not-too-favored relative. Not coincidently, 35 years is about the minimum age at which we could reasonably expect a practice administrator to be ready to run a challenging practice. At 55 years and above, we typically see both surgeons and administrators at the height of their prowess. Score yourself on this key factor (which, obviously, will improve somewhat automatically with age!).

Score: 0 1 2

#2. An Energizing Spirit

Most people enjoy movies, concerts, and stage plays, in part because they are so energizing. After 2 hours you walk back out onto the street more pumped and powerful than when you entered the theater. In a tangible and nonmanipulative sense, powerful and effective administrators are like effective performers. They add positive energy to each person in the practice. Where are you as an administrator on this trait?

Score: 0 1 2

#3. Close-to-Perfect Performance Standards, but Still Human

Ophthalmology likes to pride itself on having a perfect performance standard. This is, of course, something of an urban myth. Half of all ophthalmologists perform below average surgery and half work in below average practices. However, the vast majority of both lay staff and providers strive for perfection. The best administrators are infected early in their careers by this institutional, ophthalmological striving for perfection, while tempering this with the knowledge that human staff will often fall short of this goal. How (reasonably) perfectionistic are you?

Score: 0 1 2

#4. Communication Excellence in All Forms and Situations

The especially effective administrators are lucid. They capture and convey both facts and moods in the fewest words possible. Whether writing, speaking, or even sending nonverbal signals, they make themselves clear to others. They help team members who see things differently get on the same page. They translate the board's wishes to the rank and file and the rank-and-file staff's concerns back up the chain of command. How do you perform in this area?

Score: 0 1 2

#5. Numeracy: A Visceral Feel for and Enjoyment of Numbers

Effective practice leaders ask objective questions obliging numeric answers. Not "How's it going in billing this week?" But rather "What percentage of our open accounts are still out over 90 days?" They have as memorized and integrated a grasp of the practice's key performance indictors as surgeons do of their favorite patient's latest glaucoma statistics. They know when the numbers are favorable. They know when the numbers are way off and corrective action is needed. And most importantly, like a great physician, they know their own limitations. When they are mystified by an adverse figure, they seek advice. How are you, numbers-wise?

Score: 0 1 2

#6. Relationships With the Owners as a Trusted Peer-Collaborator, Not Minion

This attribute is a two-way street. An administrator, to be effective, must have the board's enduring confidence. But, so too, must the board—and especially the managing partner—enjoy the confidence of the company's lay leader. Weak boards kill administrative performance faster and more completely than weak administrators can kill practices. If you think your board may be disappointed in your current performance, ask yourself, "How much of this is due to fair and measurable performance gaps on my part, and how much of it is due to just a board-based gap in communication or lack of respect for the role of the administrator?"

Score: 0 1 2

#7. A Builder of Alignment Between Owners, Managers, and Staff

Imagine dropping a fistful of toothpicks on an empty table, with each toothpick representing one member of your practice. Would the resulting disarray represent your practice as it stands today, a jumble, or is everyone aligned and heading in the same direction—as the toothpicks looked before you took them out of the box? Great administrators are natural "aligners." They like to straighten and line things up. They articulate a few chief goals and help to align everyone to make progress in that one direction.

Score: 0 1 2

#8. Multifocal: The Ability to See Both the Big Picture and the Tiniest Details

Because eye surgeons deal in such minutia, it's only natural that they should be most comfortable when they are working with lay managers who are similarly obsessive. Such attention to detail is necessary but not sufficient in superior administrators. In addition to picking out the granular details, the effective manager can stand back and see how all the grains make up a beach, a boulder, or a sandstone cliff.

Score: 0 1 2

#9. Excellent Middle Manager Selection, Training, and Delegation

The biggest rookie mistake of young administrators is to not sufficiently develop and lean on their mid-level staff. In the truly great ophthalmology practices of the planet, the administrator, executive director, or CEO could be absent for a month, and the department heads would keep their companies humming.

Score: 0 1 2

#10. A Company-Wide Role Model as a Calm, Efficient, Intensely Hard Worker

The best practice leaders are the first to arrive and the last to leave. They walk just a bit faster down the hall than everyone else. When you watch them thinking about a problem, there's a furrowed-brow intensity that rivals the country's leading surgeons ... and then a smile when they've got an answer. They multitask. They remember last year's conversations as well as they remember last week's. Like the best surgeons, they embody a relaxed intensity. Maddeningly, they are almost always right.

Score: 0 1 2

Now add up your score. With 10 different attributes, and with up to two points each, there's a maximum score of 20. There is no objective scale that compares you to others, but this summary score can be a valuable personal baseline of your fitness and can help point out areas to improve. And don't be too hard on yourself if you've scored yourself in the low teens or even lower. Some of the sharpest administrators we know are their own worst critics. It's interesting to have your managing partner or an administrator-peer complete this same survey about you so you can compare the two scores.

Total score:

And then what? Consider focusing on just one or two of the areas above and write down your commitment to an improvement plan, such as:

The board and I are not on the same page about where our practice is heading in the future. I will work on #7 and my recently reduced sense of partnership with the board. I'll redouble my personal efforts and enlist the help of our most progressive partner, with whom I have the best relationship. I will harness her enthusiasm to help me win the rest of the owners over to the idea of expanding to a second office location.

A version of this chapter originally appeared in *Ophthalmic Leadership: A Practical Guide for Physicians, Administrators, and Teams, Second Edition*. For more information about *Ophthalmic Leadership*, please visit www.routledge.com.

CHAPTER 2

The Role of Assertiveness in Effective Practice Administration

New Yorkers, by reputation, are fast-talking, assertive and easily annoyed. I fit right in.
—Jane Pauley

You have the right to say no without feeling guilty.
—Manuel J. Smith

If liberty means anything at all, it means the right to tell people what they don't want to hear.
—George Orwell

One definition of the word "assertive" is "showing a confident and forceful personality," which is something everyone in a leadership position should reasonably strive to achieve, right?

But what does it mean to be *effectively* assertive in the generally genteel, non-confrontational word of ophthalmology? It's a question of balance. The key is to be assertive, as the definition of the word describes, while also being gentle … and not just mastering the first three letters of the word "assertive." Being an "ass" instead of being gently assertive makes you very ineffective and quickly alienates everyone you need on your side. Hotheads, bullies, and asses rarely go very far in this business.

Wohl C, Pinto JB. *UP: Taking Ophthalmic Administrators and Their Management Teams to the Next Level of Skill, Performance, and Career Satisfaction, Second Edition* (pp 13-15). © 2021 Taylor & Francis Group.

Here are three specific examples from settings that may be a lot like yours today. They come from practices we've worked with in the last couple of years:

1. Imagine you work in a solo practice, with very low profit margins, just 30%. There are two reasons for this low performance. First, your surgeon loves new technology and buys several new and expensive "toys" every year that he then rarely uses at a level needed to cover their cost. Second, he also insists on your staffing his clinic with four full-time techs, even though he sees only 35 patients a day and works three clinic days a week (which by the way is about 50% overstaffed). Being assertive is when you say, "You and I are both concerned about our low level of profitability. As a surgeon, you are making a lot less than your peers. If you are willing to work another half day a week and let me right-size tech staffing, we can give you a $175,000 annual pay raise."
2. Last year, the practice you manage only grew a disappointing 1% in patient visits and collections. The main reason for this was that several highly productive surgeons in your practice took eight or more weeks of vacation, when they would normally take just five. Your board delivers the mandate, "We want you and your managers to deliver at least a 5% growth rate." Being assertive is when you say, "I think this revenue boost is feasible under two conditions. First, we boost provider staffing to a level needed to see 5% more patients than we see today, and second, we double our annual marketing budget to $120,000. With these resources, I know our practice can grow at your desired rate."
3. You are the manager of a two-surgeon oculoplastics practice. Dr. Arthur generates $800,000 in annual collections. Dr. Barbara generates $1.5 million in collections. Why the difference? Because Dr. B has been in practice for 10 years longer than Dr. A, her fellowship emphasized elective/cosmetic work, she takes little vacation time, and she works one more clinic day per week than Dr. A. Dr. A comes to you, complaining about his low numbers. Being assertive is when you say, "I agree that it would be great for you, and great for the practice, to enhance your productivity. Unfortunately, I can't control any of the most important variables that make your partner twice as busy as you are. But I do think that if we three sit down together we could come up with a corrective action plan that could get you busier. If you're ready to do that—and to follow-through with the actions under your personal control—I'm ready to call a meeting."

Notice in these examples that the administrators are not being snarky or passive aggressive or nonspecific. They are confident and positive. They are mustering facts and data to back up their assertiveness.

Would you like to do the same? Here are seven Assertiveness Rules for you to consider:

1. The only boards and bosses worth working for are those who applaud your tendency to speak up for what you believe to be true and in the company's best interests. You can't be effectively assertive, much less professionally happy, in an environment with insecure or defensive practice owners who would prefer that you cower.
2. Management is not merely theater (although acting skills are helpful). Being more <u>assertive</u> obliges you to be more <u>certain</u> about your position. Stridently asserting something later found to be wrong is a great way to blow up your career.
3. Assertiveness is a poor substitute for competency. Seek first to become competent before becoming assertive. This is especially true in the areas of finance and benchmarking and in tracking key performance indicators. Know your numbers cold.
4. Know your audience and be proportionate in your style and tone. Some people you supervise (and work for) will get your assertiveness message when you raise an eyebrow. Others need a two-by-four. Both approaches should be in your toolbox as a leader.
5. The most effective assertiveness is the kind you bring forward on behalf of the overall company and the people in it, not just your own ego or interests. Try not to stand alone, make sure you have at least one equally assertive advocate supporting you, the practice's administrator if you are a mid-level supervisor, or the managing partner if you manage the overall practice.
6. Balance assertiveness with acquiescence. Yielding to others generously when appropriate gives you more credibility when you have to be periodically forceful. All the same, try to be consistent in your level of assertiveness, cycling from warrior to wimp and back again will confuse the troops and the board members alike.
7. Always be fair. People will work for—and thrive under—the toughest bosses on the planet if these bosses are also perceived to be fair.

CHAPTER 3

Getting More Done

Organization, Prioritization, Delegation, and Time Management

You have to decide what your highest priorities are and have the courage—pleasantly, smilingly, nonapologetically—to say "no" to other things. And the way to do that is by having a bigger "YES" burning inside.
—Stephen Covey

No man goes before his time—unless the boss leaves early.
—Groucho Marx

The holy trinity of great practice administration and management are organization, prioritization, and delegation. These three skills are interdependent. If just one of these skills is weak, the remaining two skills have a hard time standing on their own and you will find it challenging to thrive as a leader.

Taken together, when these three skills are present in equal measure, others will say things like, "Wow! You are great at time management!" But great time management is just the outer manifestation of organizing, prioritizing, and delegating.

Wohl C, Pinto JB. *UP: Taking Ophthalmic Administrators and Their Management Teams to the Next Level of Skill, Performance, and Career Satisfaction, Second Edition* (pp 17-24). © 2021 Taylor & Francis Group.

Organization

A common manifestation of being disorganized is to be repeatedly wasting time to search for filed documents, whether paper or electronic, and to touch (or open) documents multiple times before taking action. You may find yourself opening an email, reading it, getting stuck on what to do with it … and then repeating these actions. A more tangible, visible manifestation of disorganization may be present in your personal office. Are you a "filer" or a "piler?" Do you have stacks (on your desk AND on the floor?) Do you move paper around but never seem to finish the task or file it, so you have to handle it again later?

Or perhaps you are the kind of executive who is really good at organizing and reorganizing a project, but have trouble making significant forward progress on it? Or you fix a problem temporarily (to save time in the moment), but the fix is not enduring.

There are hundreds of ways to organize tasks, projects, and all of your responsibilities. To get you started and focused on discovering the ways that will work for you, this chapter includes basic guidelines and a few samples to try. In Chapter 8, you will find sample departmental checklists. The lists below focus on individual performance.

It is common to hear from administrators and managers that feeling overwhelmed and stressed is a barrier to being as organized as they would like to be. And it may feel counterintuitive to spend even more time making lists!

But there are definitely long-term benefits to the short-term inconveniences of finding new ways to reorganize your own workload. And once you can stop feeling reactive to issues and start being more proactive, you will have time for both daily tasks as well as higher-level management responsibilities, such as financial trend analysis and strategic planning. Here are a few great places to begin for administrators and mid-level managers alike:

Tidy Up

1. It's hard to feel organized when your workspace is a mess.
2. Block out an appropriate spring cleaning session in your calendar. If you run a larger organization, this may take a full weekend and involve the assistance of support staff.
3. Throw out everything you no longer use or need: old textbooks, old project files, piles of aging periodicals, etc.
4. Move from your desk to your employees' desks anything that they should be doing for you. Ditto for any projects that can reasonably be outsourced (like tasking your compliance consulting firm with a chart audit rather than taking this critical/technical task on yourself).
5. Except for a couple of family photos and related treasures, push everything out of your office that doesn't relate to your job.
6. At this point, if your housekeeping staff have been cleaning around your piles, do a deep cleaning.

7. Make sure you have clearly visible in and out baskets (even if you work in a small practice and you are your own personal assistant trafficking your out box).
8. Make sure your phone unit is of a type and location that serves your purpose. Many administrators find that having a Bluetooth/hands-free unit is the only way to go.
9. Have one defined location for less urgent reading (business periodicals and the like); when the stack gets too large, take it home and finish it on the weekend or toss it out … don't let it climb up the wall and spawn adjacent stacks.
10. Make sure your desk is large enough, especially if your natural tendency is to pile rather than file. Although computers have streamlined the paper chase, the managers of especially large practices have to manage an irreducible volume of paper.
11. Make sure your chair is comfortable … or better yet, arrange a standing desk for greater workplace health.

Inventory Your Workload

Some executives will say, "I've go so much to do, I don't have time to make a list of my tasks." Consider this: If you don't have time to inventory your tasks, how on earth do you have enough time to actually do them?

1. First, make sure you have a written position description. This is likely to be a generalized document, not too granular. Look this document over, make any obvious changes needed, and then set it aside for the moment.
2. Next, gathering together all of your sticky notes and scratch paper reminders, make a list (on paper, on a Microsoft Excel or Word screen, or in a dedicated task management program like Outlook) of everything that needs to be done and by when. At the outset, don't get too picky about organizing this list into categories … just push out a master, stream-of-consciousness to-do list.
3. Next, try to apply some organization to the list. There is no one way to do this. You may choose to divide it into functional areas (eg, finance, operations, quality assurance) or arrange your master to-do list based on when things are due.
4. Now that you've organized the work (and perhaps feel better having tossed away the 35 sticky notes you were using), reorganize these tasks in priority order. Remember that if everything is a priority, nothing is a priority. Force yourself to choose, using an A, B, C or similar grading system from most to least urgent.
5. Examine and think about your master list more closely. Is your list so massive it signals that you need to delegate more avidly or hire an assistant? Are there low-priority items that can simply be discarded because they really don't add proportional value?
6. The master list you have created should now become a permanent part of your organizational system, and it should be updated from time to time (weekly in some settings, monthly in others).

7. Now, how do we tackle the work? You certainly can't do all of the work on your master list in a single day or week. The most effective executives use a master list like this to create their daily task list. Here are a few simple rules about creating and using this daily list:
   a. Update or rewrite your daily task list at the end of every day for the following day (don't figure out what you are going to do after you arrive in the office in the morning).
   b. Make sure the task list is realistic. You are not going to get very far down your list if it's a day full of meetings.
   c. Start each day with the *task that is most important.* This may mean it's also the most gruesome and difficult task of the day ... no matter ... do it first and get it over with.
   d. Fight procrastination. The most fortunate managers have good internal discipline: They stick to their diet, go to the gym, and stay on task with their to-do lists. Everyone else needs an external source of discipline. This can be a personal assistant to keep you on track (most administrators in practices with $8 million of revenue and higher routinely have such a position). In smaller settings, a timer may help: Select a task. Determine how much time you have to complete the task. Set a count-down timer (such as a kitchen timer or digital watch). And then let the timer be a source of external discipline to help push you along.
8. Once you are more organized, it will be easier to delegate some of the work. It may be a whole project or just a piece of one, but push beyond your comfort level to allow others to help you do your work.
9. Finally, compare your master task list to your written position description. Do they synch? If not, why not? Decide what you need to do about that, and whether you (and your practice board) are being realistic about your formal scope of work.

Further Organizational Pearls

- Ask: Am I allotting the right amount of time for each task? Is there a skill I am missing that delays task completion? Why do I misjudge the time it takes to complete tasks?
- Ask: Am I the only one who can be doing this task or can I delegate it now or in the future? Prepare a running list for immediate delegation or future delegation opportunity—perhaps once someone else is educated, the project becomes more mature or you've hired someone else, then you can include it in their role, etc.
- Ask: Do I really need to check email every 15 minutes, or would it be more efficient to respond at a few set times each day? This approach could provide the time and space I need to focus without interruption and allow me to control my work flow.
- Ask: Am I harnessing the potential $1+1=3$ impact of working more closely with my managing partner and department heads, to help me prioritize and off-load appropriate projects?
- Ask: With everything else on my plate, am I getting out of my office enough (ideally several times a day) to observe clinic flow and talk to a couple of staff and patients about how we're doing today?

Prioritization

Everything is not critically important, at least not at the same time, even though on some days it may feel like it, and every item on your task list is written in red ink with a star next to it. Your doctors may be tempted to say, "Everything we do in this practice is a top priority," but that will not be executable in any reasonable way. If everything is declared a priority, nothing is a priority.

Prioritizing determines what is most important and subsequently what you (and the practice) want to be spending more time working on, rather than haphazardly spending time on whatever presents itself. It helps the organization stay aligned when every department's work is a concerted effort toward the same major practice goals.

Prioritizing is a largely subjective activity, a "feelings thing." But you can artificially and helpfully try to objectify the process of prioritizing your work flow.

The most common measurements in business are economic. What is the potential bottom line impact of each of your action items? Clearly, its more financially critical that you recredential with an important third-party payer than talk to painting vendors about trim colors. But because your practice is more than a business, you may decide to prioritize your work list using some other values including:

- Quality of care: What best impacts patient safety and outcomes?
- Reputation: What tasks will increase our status in the community?
- Staff considerations: What priorities on my to-do list will have the greatest impact on workplace enjoyment and staff tenure?

The Pareto Principle, more commonly known as the *80/20 rule*, reminds us that 20% of your actions will provide 80% of the results. So plan your action carefully. Prioritize project work by scheduling time on your calendar. Don't leave your days unstructured so you are squeezing the most important tasks into randomly unused spots in your day. Be self-disciplined about your time management by prioritizing your work.

Delegation

Delegation is a learned skill. As children we are taught to take responsibility for our actions. To clean up our own messes. To do our own school work. But responsibility in the business world doesn't mean you have to do everything by yourself. As an administrator or department manager, you will appropriately be held responsible for the outcome of an assignment, but, more often than not, it will be a team effort, under your direction and guidance.

The need for you to delegate, and your ability to do so, will vary depending on the size of your practice and your position in it. Your ability to delegate will also change over the course of your career. With (hopefully) growing seniority in a (hopefully) growing practice, you will wake up one day and wonder why you are still sorting the mail.

It is common for us to hear from the administrators for whom we work, "I delegate everything I possibly can." But when we start to probe the details together ... not so true. It can be comforting to hold on to familiar, even fun, tasks you have been completing yourself for years. But it is not practical or efficient. Nor is it a service to your practice or your career.

Here are questions and concepts to consider, whether you are an administrator or a mid-level manager:

- Am I delegating appropriately? How can I improve this skill? Begin by referencing your position description. Your personal responsibilities and duties must be clear (and agreed upon by your supervisor) before you will be comfortable delegating work.
- Being confident about your duties can also (sometimes subtly) impact the way you delegate work. You don't want to be apologizing for delegating. If you apologize (eg, Jenn, I'm really sorry to have to ask you do this for me, but I don't have the time), the designee will not feel as responsible for the work product as if it were one of their own duties.
- List your primary responsibilities and ask if they can only be done by you? Partially by you? Entirely by someone else on your team?
- It is important to acknowledge you are ultimately responsible for the completion of all of your designated responsibilities. As the saying goes, "The buck stops here." It is your responsibility to make sure an assignment to a staffer is clear. Be specific with instructions and expectations.
- Follow up to make sure the assignment was not only completed but completed properly. If it is the first time you are delegating a new task, check early progress on the assignment so there is time to redirect your staffer and avoid generating discouragement or annoyance with your poor instructions.
- If the assignment is not completed with acceptable performance, remind yourself, "It is my responsibility to teach and counsel the employee how to do it better next time." Don't get frustrated and go back to doing it yourself. Provide yourself and your employee with an opportunity to improve and grow professionally.

Bonus Tool: Using a Gantt Chart

A Gantt Chart (named for Henry Gantt in the early 1900s) is another way to organize complex, multipart projects that take place over several months. Examples include building projects, hiring new doctors, and adding new service lines like LASIK or dry eye treatment. The simplified example here shows steps to launch a new practice. Modify it to fit your practice needs the next time you have a large project to supervise.

Sample Practice Startup Gantt Chart

	J	F	M	A	M	J	J	A	S	O	N	D
Review personal issues: Budget, time commitment, risk tolerance, options	X											
Commit to launch a new practice		X										
Unwind existing employment/ partnership		X	X	X	X							
Write business plan and pro forma		X	X	X								
Secure accountant, attorney, consultants, banker, insurance agent, designers, etc		X	X	X	X							
Apply for and secure financing, line of credit, leases			X	X	X	X						
Select the form of business (eg, LLC, LLP)			X	X	X							
Choose a practice name			X	X	X							
Establish legal entity				X	X	X	X					
Provider numbers, credentialing, panel access work, etc.					X	X	X	X	X	X	X	X
Outreach to referral sources					X	X	X	X	X	X	X	X
Decide on location and secure lease					X	X	X	X				
Space planning						X	X	X	X			
Select and purchase furnishings/ equipment							X	X	X	X	X	
Select phone/fax/cable/ communications							X	X	X	X		
Practice management and electronic health record systems							X	X	X	X		

(continued)

Sample Practice Startup Gantt Chart (continued)

	J	F	M	A	M	J	J	A	S	O	N	D
Alarm, security cameras, etc.							X	X	X			
Signs and signage								X	X	X		
Select and employ administrator/ office manager								X	X	X	X	
Select IT platform, install, train								X	X	X	X	X
Build-out and occupancy permit								X	X	X	X	
Cleaning service									X	X	X	
Prepare marketing communications materials									X	X	X	
Staff uniforms, name tags, orientation, etc.									X	X		
Hire initial staff										X	X	
Open the new office												X
Open house events												X
Ongoing operations polishing												X

CHAPTER 4

Prioritizing Your To-Do List

A major part of successful living lies in the ability to put first things first. Indeed the reason most major goals are not achieved is that we spend our time doing second things first.
—Robert J. McKain

Guessing is cheap; guessing wrong is expensive.
—Chinese proverb

Surgeons learn early in their training to triage—addressing big medical problems first and small ones later. And yet, somehow, too little of this lesson is applied when doctors and managers are running their practice businesses. Everything can be flagged as a priority, which is a little like a doctor treating a patient's shattered orbit and toe blister at the same time. Learning how to quickly and effectively prioritize business tasks is at the heart of great practice management.

We all pay lip service to prioritization. The surgeon-owner asks the administrator, "What are you working on now, Susan?" "Plans for the new satellite office," Susan replies. And yet, when she continues down the hall to her office, Susan faces a whiteboard with a list of 26 urgent tasks, none of which is really number one.

Practices, managing partners, and administrators who thrive develop a system to nominate the most important tasks and communicate these priorities up and down the organization.

Applying Stephen Covey's advice, it's best to tend to the nonurgent/important items before turning to urgent (and only seemingly important) ones.

But the contemporary demands on practice leaders encourage all of us to either address the "on fire" issues (which could have been prevented with earlier attention), or worse, to put first efforts every day into those things that are either easy to check off your list or fun to do, but not necessarily priorities. By the end of the day, the truly important tasks can be left untouched. Again.

Good and bad prioritization habits are part of each practice's culture. We see practices where everyone diligently pursues the most important priorities first … and practices where the opposite is true.

What's the culture of your practice? Do you apply major attention to major items? Is procrastination called out or overlooked by your board with or by you with your management team? Are blown deadlines blown off, or is there an appropriate, adverse consequence for not getting your agreed-upon tasks done on time?

Prioritization is so important, and fundamental to success, it's something best periodically relaunched formally at the board level and then refreshed once again down the ranks. Doing this creates a culture of shared urgencies.

Business prioritization is perhaps more art than science, something that the most fortunate of us stumble upon for ourselves rather than by learning an effective system. But all effective executives eventually find what works best for them. If you want to speed up the process of learning how to better prioritize, what follows is a systematic approach, abstracted from the best habits we see in our travels around the country and the world:

1. First, let's discuss <u>structure</u>. Examine your current list, no matter how ugly. Ask:
    a. What's the format of your list? Consistency here is as important as what physical tool you use. Some perfectly excellent managers manage their to-do list on 3 × 5 cards, others on a yellow tablet, or, like most today, in a Microsoft Word file or Outlook task list. All of these can work, but work best if used consistently.
    b. Do you have a system that flags true priorities? This can be A, B, C or 1 through 5, or even a simple asterisk.
    c. Do you review and update your task list at appropriate intervals? Obsessively editing your list several times a day is not an effective use of your time—but neither is checking your list weekly. Some of the most effective ophthalmic executives we know make it a habit to examine their to-do list closely twice a day, once at the start of the workday as a reminder of the priorities, and once at the end of the day, when the next day's priorities are flagged.
    d. Are the right time frames covered? Your current to-do list should probably not be bogged down with tasks you won't tackle until next quarter.
    e. Are all of the tasks on your list really yours? Or do you clog up your to-do list with the actions for which others are responsible, simply to ensure you haven't forgotten what you delegated?

2. After considering the structure and content of your action list, let's turn to function. The whole reason for having an action list is to stay on task with the priorities of your company. Do you know what these are? Surprisingly, fewer than 5% of practices have a formal, written strategic plan. But even in the absence of a plan, your practice's leadership team should at least have a punch list of longer-term strategic priorities, each of which should match up with one or more actions on your to do-list. Here's an example:

Sample Strategic Priority	Sample Tactical Actions
Grow practice revenue 7% annually	• Hire an advertising agency to help boost new patient volumes • Audit recall systems in the practice
Improve cataract surgical outcomes	• Secure surgeon buy-in to measure individual outcomes • Agree on a methodology to measure these outcomes
Complete a succession plan to replace a retiring senior partner with a new partner-track associate	• Draw up employment and prospective partnership buy-in terms • Engage a recruiting firm

3. And last comes discipline. Make sure you apply sufficient energy and focus. The best list-making in the world is for naught unless you take action on your action list. Here are a few pearls from the most diligent administrators we know:
   a. As a mechanic pal once said, "When you lift up the hood do something easy first—it gets your confidence up." You, too, may feel more accomplished if you complete one or two easy things first. This may give you confidence and boost momentum.
   b. Alternately, if you are the procrastinating type, you may find it most effective each day to tackle first the most gruesome of your projects.
   c. Don't forget to cross each completed item off your list (or change the color of that line item on your electronic list). Celebrating each completed task acts as a small reward to propel you through the day.
   d. The fastest way to plow through a to-do list is to *not* do some of the things at all. Is there anything on the list that can be eliminated altogether?
   e. Review your task list for items you can delegate. Does everything on the list require your personal attention, or can some of it be distributed inside the practice or outsourced?
   f. Don't be too harsh on yourself. An ophthalmic executive's task list is never completely checked off. In most settings, you have to live with practical limits on how many big picture tasks you can be pursuing at one time. Most of each day will often be spent on general practice operations, obliging that some of your daily to-do list will be carried forward to the next day, no matter the priority.

Quick Start: How to Assess if You Help or Hinder Prioritizing in Your Practice or Department

Being realistic about what it takes to perform the assignments you give your staff (or yourself) is the first step to successfully identifying what should be prioritized in your practice.

Here is a short list to help you and your managers evaluate how carefully you are prioritizing projects and tasks. Once you identify where improvement is needed, create a written plan to document the steps you want to take to enhance this skill.

- I listen to and carefully consider manager and employee feedback about workloads and duties throughout the practice.
- I know how to judge whether I have realistic expectations of employees or there are individual performance issues to be addressed. (And if I am not sure, I will investigate and learn.)
- I know how to assess and then guide employees who don't say "no" to any assignments but then express feeling overwhelmed or frustrated.
- I (or "we" as a management team) clearly express goals and expectations in our practice so our employees are informed and can prioritize their own work appropriately.

CHAPTER 5

Strengthen Your Career and Practice With Accountability Tools

A river cuts through rock, not because of power,
but because of persistence.
—Jim Watkins

It is not only what we do, but also what we do not do,
for which we are accountable.
—Molière

Accountability is the measure of a leader's height.
—Jeffrey Benjamin

Managing the business of medicine and practicing medicine are in many ways symmetric. To diagnose patient problems, doctors gather information, make a treatment decision, suggest treatment options, and monitor the results, and then repeat the process if the outcome is not satisfactory. Administrators follow a similar pattern to identify and solve practice problems.

Patients hold doctors accountable for their actions. If their problems are not resolved, they return. If they are unhappy with their medical treatment or the way the staff treated them, they find a new doctor or at least write a poor review online.

Wohl C, Pinto JB. *UP: Taking Ophthalmic Administrators and Their Management Teams to the Next Level of Skill, Performance, and Career Satisfaction, Second Edition* (pp 29-34). © 2021 Taylor & Francis Group.

How can administrators and the management team hold each other and the rest of the staff accountable in your practice? Making yourselves accountable for all significant functions in your practice is a keystone to a successful and well-managed organization.

Accountability, as defined by *Merriam-Webster*, is "an obligation or willingness to accept responsibility or to account for one's actions." Surgeons are trained to be hypervigilant and hold themselves responsible for patient outcomes. The majority of surgeons are proud to share their excellent outcome data and will lose a few nights' sleep over a rare complication. The concept of accountability is pounded deeply into the best ophthalmologists.

Why, then, is it so difficult for many ophthalmic business owners to hold their management, employee doctors, or each other, as owners, accountable? Or to allow their administrator and management team to hold employees less responsible for their actions than would be optimal?

We think it starts with the "ophthalmic personality." Ophthalmologists tend to be nonconfrontational by nature. (You may have noticed this if you have worked for other specialists: in our experience, orthopedists and neurosurgeons are often more assertive and many love confrontation.) Physicians, in our observation, tend to pass this gentle personality down to employees. Before you know it, the practice culture that evolves can be less confrontational than is helpful in pure business terms. And, human nature being what it is, a nonconfrontational environment has a much lower level of accountability.

Less gets done, and it gets done to a lower standard. Accountability is the key to practice performance in all dimensions. Practices that consistently hold all staff accountable find that problems are solved faster and easier. New problems and adverse trends can be identified promptly when there is one person who owns each dimension of practice performance.

Here are some examples of accountability standards and tools; some are in every practice and some may be missing in your setting:

- Patient records: This is a fundamental accountability document in medicine. As the old saying goes, "If it's not in the chart, it wasn't done." Charts hold doctors accountable to patients, payers, and peers alike.
- Checklists: An increasing number of practices are developing formal checklists for each department. These can be monthly, weekly, or even daily, and help managers be more accountable to their company.
- Documented, objective, quarterly goals for administrators and managers that set clear expectations, define success, and provide the basis for understanding why goals may not be completed.
- Written performance appraisals for all employees that specify goals and the suggested steps needed to meet them. Ideally the appraisals are oriented around each employee's work anniversary date and any salary increase is tied to performance and not the outdated cost-of-living increase.
- For physicians, a board-approved code of conduct helps set standards that identify which behaviors are acceptable or not in your practice, like arriving for clinic on time or following written care pathways predetermined by practice leadership.

Creating a culture of accountability takes a full commitment from the management team. And as an administrator, it is vital that you get the support of physician-leaders in your practice.

• • •

Here are several accountability tools that can help maintain high standards for patient care and practice management.

Tool #1: Strategic Goals

Strategy and tactics are often confused. Strategic planning for your practice answers questions (over time frames of 3 years or longer) such as "How fast do we want to grow?" "What services should we add?" "How many MDs and ODs will we employ?" "What's our succession plan?" In comparison, tactics are actions deployed in the service of tactics, you might ramp up marketing activities if your strategic goals are to grow at a faster pace. Written strategic goals allow administrators and managers alike to be more accountable to (and successful at accomplishing) the board's business ambitions.

Tool #2: Benchmarking

Just as ophthalmologists are accustomed to comparing one patient's intraocular pressure to normal pressures, and comparing a patient's visual acuity to the standard of 20/20, practice managers should similarly be able to compare internal benchmark data to national standards.

There are approximately 50 common practice benchmarks used in ophthalmology to compare normative values to your own practice statistics. Examples include profit margin, staff labor productivity, facility utilization, and surgical density. (A complete list can be found in *John Pinto's Little Green Book of Ophthalmology, Sixth Edition*, published by SLACK Incorporated.)

The administrator is accountable to the board of directors to ensure that the practice is hitting these normative benchmarks or, if it is not, that a corrective action plan is in place.

Tool #3: Action Grid

An action grid, which is one example of an accountability document, is comparable to a medical record, where history, diagnosis, and progress are documented—but it applies to the business side of a practice. This sample document contains four columns. The first column lists the specific task or project; the second column identifies who is responsible for completing the task. The third column posts the deadline, and the fourth column holds progress notes and status updates. The progress note section most importantly helps keep all managers and doctors who have access to this shared document informed about how each project is coming along. Imagine how much time is saved by the management team reading the update notes prior to a meeting, rather than sitting in the meeting while each person speaks about every project. You will find instructions for developing your own action grid at the end of this chapter.

Tool #4: Checklists

Checklists are another great written aid to help your managers monitor task completion in their departments. Establishing a checklist of the necessary tasks to be completed on a daily or weekly basis keeps the staff organized and goal oriented. The department or site manager can require the completed checklists be initialed and submitted at the end of the week. Imagine the time this saves compared to each manager having to verbally check in with multiple staff. Or more often, managers find out after the fact that tasks were not completed and a problem then needs solving. Checklists help managers and administrators be proactive rather than reactive.

Tool #5: Accountable Communication

We will discuss accountable communication extensively in Chapter 6, so we won't go into more detail here. But here is an important reminder: Delaying a necessary discussion rarely improves a problem situation. We most often hear, after nudging clients forward, "I sure wish I had done that sooner."

Tool #6: Performance Appraisals

Performance appraisals can help guide both employee and manager by stating clearly how individual goal-setting ties into overall practice goals. Staffers have the opportunity to grow professionally and be more productive when made aware of their strengths and weaknesses at least annually. If they are not meeting expectations, management has this opportunity to develop a formal corrective action plan.

Expectations are best served when described in measurable ways. Instead of saying, "We want you to become a better biller," the manager can say, "You are posting 100 charges per day. In the next 90 days, we would like you to post 150 charges per day." This sets an objective standard on which future performance reviews can be based.

In the same regard, telling a doctor, "You need to be friendlier to patients," is not measurable in a way that helps the doctor improve. A better approach is to conduct a patient satisfaction survey and then provide specific ideas and measures for improvement.

The challenge of holding doctors, managers—and yourself!—accountable can be uncomfortable in the moment, but it is profoundly rewarding over time. Using accountability documents adds a measure of discipline and streamlines the time you spend following up on what has yet to be accomplished.

Managing a practice with a core value of holding all individuals accountable for their work not only increases work productivity and tempo, but aligns individual and departmental priorities with overall practice priorities.

Developing and Using an Action Grid in Your Practice

A cornerstone of optimal practice management is an accountability document memorializing all of the larger, open projects in the company. This document is analogous to a patient chart that helps doctors be more accountable for the clinical care they provide.

Each practice manager has a personal preference for the form of this document. Some like a complex, dedicated program like Microsoft Project, but a simple action grid generally suffices and eliminates having to teach people a new program. Following is a sample grid (and grid rules). Your grid can be easily created and maintained in Microsoft Word or Excel.

Instructions

1. The grid is only to be used as a log for larger projects and initiatives. It should not be used for standing items (eg, "complete staff performance reviews") or for small matters that are quickly cleared. For a sense of the threshold an item should reach to be on the grid, it is unlikely that a managing partner or administrator would have more than 5 to 10 open items or that a department head would have more than four open items.
2. Consider using a priority code (eg, A, B, C) to aid communication and agreement on the priorities.
3. The action grid should be on the shared drive and available to all providers and managers.
4. Action items should be in subject-predicate format and be stated clearly enough that anyone reading them would be able to discern when the action is indeed accomplished:
   a. Not this: "Electronic health record (EHR) development"
   b. This: "Select an agreed-upon new EHR vendor, establish an implementation calendar, and go live with 100% of providers using."

5. Action items should be clustered by owner (ie, all of Mary's items are next to each other). This will facilitate the grid's use as the management committee's meeting agenda … "As you can see I have four open items. The first three are self-explanatory, and we are making good progress, but I need the committee's input on my fourth item, where I'm stuck."
6. There should be only one person responsible for each line item in most cases.
7. The deadline column should be filled in with a specific date ("April 23") not "5 weeks" or "Q4."
8. Progress notes for each open item should be updated (by its owner—not the administrator, office manager, or executive assistant) 48 hours in advance of every management committee meeting, and a copy should be printed out for each attendee at the meeting. All attendees should read their copy before coming to the meeting and be prepared to present to the group on their open items.
9. The updated grid should be emailed to any owner who will not be present at the management committee meeting. All owners should have open access to this file, and even if they are not active in a management role, they can check on progress with items of importance to them.
10. If an item is approved but tabled for now, enter the "tabled to ____" date in the deadline column so it's not lost.
11. Completed items should be moved to the bottom of the file or to a separate archive file. Check periodically to make sure that items once considered completed have not resurfaced.
12. On the copy you bring to a management meeting, leave a few empty lines at the bottom. In that way, if a new action item comes up, the person responsible can write in the item and the group-agreed deadline.

Action (Dated) *(Optional: Add an A, B, C priority code)*	**Who (One Person)**	**Deadline**	**Progress Notes (Dated)**
Replace worn carpet in the Smithville Office (Oct. 2) "B"	Susan	Nov. 20	Oct. 15—carpet samples reviewed and order placed Oct. 30—installation scheduled for Nov. 13 Nov. 10—date pushed back due to flood damage repair work

CHAPTER 6

Encouraging Great Communication

It is better to know some of the questions than to know all of the answers.
—James Thurber

The single biggest problem in communication is the illusion that it has taken place.
—George Bernard Shaw

The art of communication is the language of leadership.
—James Humes

Uncluttered lines of communication among managers, staff, and doctors are at the core of successful working relationships in your practice. Without reliable communication, both administrative and clinical inefficiencies arise, in turn gumming up the quality of patient care, customer service, and financial performance.

Communication, *Merriam-Webster* says, is any system of exchanging information. Incomplete communication or miscommunication in your practice masks problems and creates more work. Negative exchanges not only mask the needed communication in the moment, but may inhibit and erode future communication as well.

Wohl C, Pinto JB. *UP: Taking Ophthalmic Administrators and Their Management Teams to the Next Level of Skill, Performance, and Career Satisfaction, Second Edition* (pp 35-41).

Unfortunately, positive and appropriate communication skills don't come naturally. Communication skills are developed and honed over a lifetime, patterned after our parents, teachers, bosses, and workplace peers.

Most of us are innately poor listeners, until we get feedback from others. Most of us are defensive when we hear something about ourselves we don't like. And, most of us are inherently unpracticed at saying things in a way that is scrupulously true and direct, but still likely to be well-received by others.

Happily, you can overcome these deficits by following and practicing a few easy rules you'll learn in this chapter.

About Accountable Communication

Administrators and mid-level managers are generally excellent at being accountable—for smooth operations, cost and inventory control, patient satisfaction, and a hundred other details. If these details don't go well, they immediately feel the adverse consequences.

Accountable communication is like this, but different, in that poor communication can add up slowly over time—almost like glaucoma, a disease that can remain hidden for years—until it reaches a critical level and practice operations visibly suffer.

We talk a lot about accountable communication with clients' teams. When communication is blocked and their staff are tiptoeing around important issues, they create barriers to their own success. Communication gaps are always easier to see from the outside looking in, but you can apply the same objective outsider's approach we do by asking, "Does our team have any of these common communication skill deficits?"

Avoidance and Withholding

Accountable communication means not hiding or watering down the truth. It's being brave enough to say words you may be uncomfortable saying, and then being brave enough to hear an uncomfortable response.

When problem solving, do not withhold information or feedback for fear of hurting someone's feelings. Being direct and honest (even with the gentlest delivery) may feel uncomfortable at first. But the resulting conversation will be more productive and more real. In a business context, it increases the likelihood that the problem discussed will be solved effectively the first time, avoiding a cycle of communications friction that is not only frustrating but also costly.

We've all been in this situation. We delay confronting an employee about behavior with co-workers, hoping for improvement. The difficulty with avoidance is that it compounds problems. While you may find temporary relief in not approaching an employee about behavior issues, co-workers are increasingly angry that you are not doing anything about the problem affecting them, which reduces their respect for your leadership and decreases their performance.

Defensiveness

This is the flip side of the withholding coin. We withhold things from each other because we don't want to deal with a defensive response. Being nondefensive is a key leadership trait. It invites others to be more open with you and is as simple as saying to a disgruntled staffer, an angry doctor, or a complaining patient, "You may be right, please tell me more." Try saying these words the next time you have an angry doctor in your office.

Angry doctor: "I've had it! My patients are running 30 minutes late because the front desk can't get their paperwork done in a timely manner!"

You: "You may be right, please tell me more."

What you'll probably notice is that the angry doctor's shoulders will relax. He may go on to describe secondary causes for his running behind. He may even reflect that his delayed arrival was a part of the morning backlog. This opens up a space for you to be able to pull together a brief brainstorming session (with the doctor, involved techs, perhaps a front desk lead) to find and fix the sources of the problem.

Triangulation

This is when Dr. Bob talks to Technician Joe about his problem with Dr. Sally, instead of talking to Dr. Sally directly about the problem. It's really just another kind of withholding. It's always better to talk and solve problems directly rather than indirectly through a third person. As an administrator or department supervisor, if someone comes to you and says, "My co-worker Mary is being very difficult today!" your response should almost always be, "Have you talked to Mary about this yet?"

Ineffective Discussion

This most commonly arises when you launch a business conversation without having an advance, specific goal. As an administrator or physician, knowing the desired outcome when you launch a conversation with a staff member allows you to stay on topic and drive to a desired outcome.

This starts before you launch every important conversation. If there is a problem to solve, write out your talking points. If you want to provide positive feedback to an employee, be sure you can specifically delineate the measurable details that led them to success. This increases the odds that the desired behaviors will continue.

Ineffective Meetings

Meetings are the bane of medical practice management. Their number, frequency, and duration grow logarithmically. A practice with 30 people needs four times as much meeting time as a 15-worker practice. So, as a practice leader, one of your key missions is to run great meetings.

Important meetings held without a written agenda can signal a lack of purpose and feel frustrating and wasteful to attendees. Helping others prepare for an upcoming business meeting organizes the group and enhances outcomes. Great meeting leadership includes sending out a written agenda to all attendees at least 1 day prior to the meeting, sticking to the agenda, and sending out clear post-meeting minutes. For more on this important subject, please read Chapter 22, "How to Lead More Effective Meetings."

Lack of Follow-Up

Like a doctor, your job is to find problems, gather information, make decisions ... and then act! Even the best communication is a waste without follow-up. One of the most common staff complaints we hear is, "We've told our administrator (or managing department head) about this problem but never heard back." In both large and small practices, it's a good habit to log all meaningful suggestions and questions, and check them off as they are subsequently addressed. Even if you decide the problem raised can't be fixed (or at least fixed as quickly as a staffer may desire), it is important to provide that staff member with timely feedback about the disposition of the issue: "Alice, I'm glad you brought up the problem with our slow-moving computers. We've had our IT people look at this, and the board has decided to live with the problem until the end of this year. But by early next year we should be buying new equipment, which should really speed things up." For larger items like this, it's not only good to communicate with the one staff member who brings up an issue, but to discuss it at the next staff meeting.

Nonverbal Signals That Conflict With Your Words

Your body language and verbal tone send powerful messages. These messages may be at odds with the words you use and the intentions you have. Arms folded across your chest and scowling while verbally saying "Yes" corrupts your message in ways that you may not realize. Try to be self-observant and ask the people you trust most for feedback on the coherence between what you say and how you say it.

• • •

How do you know if communication within your practice is strong or weak? Consider these clues:

- If you are an especially effective communicator (a rare talent) people will probably point this out to you from time to time. Do they?
- Do most staff feel they can broach any subject—even difficult ones—with you and the other staff and doctors?
- Do doctors avoid the most common and challenging conversations in the boardroom: compensation modeling, capital equipment outlays, or adverse provider behavior? Why? Can you, working with your managing partner, help to break the ice and turn around this avoidance?

- Have your staff stopped making practice improvement suggestions because they never hear any feedback?
- Are you frustrated that your suggestions and orders to staff don't seem to be carried out in the way you intended?

Communication excellence comes in many forms and takes a concerted effort. Your practice's success with accountable communication starts with practice leadership setting a good example from the top.

Additional Communication

Questions and Exercises

Below are a few questions and exercises you can work though to expand your communication skills. Some of these are for your individual consideration, and some may be helpful in your setting for group discussion.

1. How often do you communicate meaningfully with your:
   a. Managing partner
   b. Solo owner or board of directors
   c. Managers
   d. Individual employees
   e. Vendors
   f. Peers (administrators from other practices)
2. For each of these contact opportunities (create one grid sheet like the one that follows for each contact), how many of the choices do you utilize with each person, and what are the benefits to expanding the ways you currently choose to communicate with each?

   Communication review with ______________________________

	Current Activity	How to Improve
Informal meetings		
Formal meetings		
Email		
Text		
Phone		
Other		

3. Your managing partner pops into your office and says, "I've got a few minutes, how's the week going?" Informal and unplanned meetings do happen. Here's how to be prepared at a moment's notice:
   a. Keep an easily accessible running list of topics to be discussed in an e-file, folder file, or noted on a pad in your desk drawer (whatever method is comfortable and quick for you). Some administrators have a file stand on their desk holding "Discuss with ____________" file folders.
   b. Use an open project list that you periodically update. On a single document you can show the project, who owns it, the deadline, and recent progress notes.
   c. Other ways I do it: ________________________________
4. For a formal, anticipated meeting:
   a. Prepare an agenda for all planned meetings. Between meetings, save time and prioritize important topics and follow-up items by keeping a running list you can refer to when making up the next agenda.
   b. Meeting minutes help keep your team marching in the same direction and improve practice productivity when each goal, responsible party, and deadline are included. For formally scheduled board meetings and the like, official meeting minutes may be the best approach. For planned meetings with only two or three attendees, a summary email following the meeting may suffice. As administrator, you get to choose if you will prepare the minutes or delegate that duty.
   c. Other ways I do it: ________________________________
5. If you suspect that you could be a better communicator but are not sure how to proceed, ask your managing partner, practice owners, and management team for feedback. "How would you score my communication skills on a 1 to 10 scale? What could I do more, less, differently to communicate more effectively?" It may feel uncomfortable to ask this, but it sends a strong message that you are open to suggestions about your performance, committed to continued professional growth, and hearing about ways to help others get their jobs done more effectively (something that you may be unknowingly impeding).
6. If you and your senior practice members are ready to take communication to the next level—and you are comfortably at a point in your communication that you can work through any temporary stress emerging from this last exercise—try this "stop-start-continue" grid.

	Stop	Start	Continue
Dr. Smith			
Dr. Jones			
Admin. Lisa			

Instructions

- This exercise is best used with small, senior workgroups, a board of directors and the administrator, or the management committee consisting of department heads, the administrator, and the managing partner. It bogs down with more than 8 to 10 people. Participants should sit around a table if possible.
- Put the names of all attendees in the left hand column of a grid sheet that looks like the example.
- Choose a moderator (it can be one of the meeting attendees or an outsider).
- Instruct participants to fill in the stop, start, continue squares for the first person. Take this one square at a time, and allow up to 1 or 2 minutes for everyone to finish each square as they go across the row.
- Then say "Now please fill in all of the remaining squares." Again, in most settings people will need about 1 minute per square to complete the exercise. Some people will be uncomfortable filling in every square (particularly the "Stop" squares). Gently encourage them to continue and fill in every square to the best of their ability.
- The resulting grid sheet will look something like this:

	Stop	Start	Continue
Dr. Smith	Arriving late in the office	Our new LASIK program	Your excellent care of patients
Dr. Jones	Allowing ad-lib work-in patients	Letting our staff scribe for you	Your attention to business details
Admin. Lisa	Letting staff get away with breaking our policies	Work on writing our strategic plan	Finishing your MBA program

- The moderator then goes around the table asking everyone in turn for their "Stops" on the first person (Dr. Smith, in this example). Each person speaking should turn to Dr. Smith and say what they have written down. In this case, Dr. Smith is not to explain or defend, but simply say, "Thank you."
- Once everyone has given their "Stops" for Dr. Smith, the moderator goes around the circle again asking for the "Starts" for Dr. Smith, and in the last round the "Continues." Then the moderator can ask Dr. Smith, "Do you have any questions or feedback?" In most settings, the individual will simply express appreciation for the honest feedback
- Move down the left side, covering the next person's stop, start, continue, and so on until every individual has given feedback on everyone at the table.

In our extensive experience with this exercise, it is not unusual for the group to emerge at the far end of what can be a somewhat draining process with a lot of barriers broken down.

Do not do this exercise without an external/neutral moderator in settings where the participants are in a longstanding conflict, or if the internal moderator is uncomfortable dealing with the emotions this exercise can evoke.

CHAPTER 7

Making the Shift From Memory to Manuals

Isn't it fortunate how selective
our recollections usually are?
—Malcolm Forbes

The palest ink lasts longer
than the most retentive memory.
—Chinese proverb

We have all forgot more than we remember.
—Thomas Fuller

This chapter is dedicated to those administrator and physician wizards whose profound memory skills allow them to keep everything about running their practice in their heads.

We'll get right to the point: *Please quit it!* A successful, growing practice will eventually overtake even the best memory skills.

A practice may grow revenue and patient volumes linearly, a few percentage points a year. But the same practice's enterprise complexity rises logarithmically. A practice that doubles in size becomes four times as complex as it was.

Wohl C, Pinto JB. *UP: Taking Ophthalmic Administrators and Their Management Teams to the Next Level of Skill, Performance, and Career Satisfaction, Second Edition* (pp 43-46).

This leads to managing partners and managers, who have been relying on memory rather than writing, hitting the wall, sometimes abruptly overwhelmed without warning as the number of moving parts and details swamps even their prodigious recall skills.

Compare this to the rest of us. Over the years, people with mere-mortal memory capacity develop hacks to stay up with an ever-evolving, convoluting practice. These hacks include:

- An operations manual used to memorialize how everything is done in the practice
- Naming conventions for computer files and passwords, rather than a random approach
- Redundancy, so that critical instructions are clearly understood by more than one person
- The abundant use of labels on storage lockers and equipment boxes, and the posting of written instructions for each piece of equipment
- Searchable files in Microsoft Word containing "idiot sheets" for how things work
- Rampant use of smartphone apps to serve as a kind of "portable brain"
- Laminated cheat-sheets for techs to keep straight what each doctor and each presenting condition needs during a work-up

Let's dive a little deeper into just one of these memory aids, albeit the largest and hardest to start—the operations manual.

One of your primal instincts as a practice leader should be to have everyone doing things the same way, right? In business, this reduces costs and errors, and it improves customer service. In ophthalmic practice, consistency saves vision and reduces malpractice exposure.

So, everyone agrees, "We should write stuff down," as a general principle for running the entire practice. When you come across something that's unsatisfactory, you should be asking, "What's our policy about this?" When there is a policy, you can follow it (or revise it). When there is no policy, you can develop one, with appropriate input from the practice's stakeholders.

But you would be surprised at how few protocols and procedures are written down in the average practice—even in quite large practices. The main impediment is a lack of time, inertia, and not knowing where to start.

Here's a simple, six-step approach to launch or enhance an operations manual for your practice. You don't have to do this alone. Even if you're a smart administrator or department head, you may not come close to knowing the granular details of how each job is done in the practice (or how it has been modified without permission since you last checked!). Instead, take this project by siege over a matter of months, and turn to staff in the trenches to do most of the work for you:

1. Gather one department team, let's say the technical department, in a 60-minute meeting. Have a whiteboard or flip chart handy and hand out pads and pens. Ask everyone to write down at least 10 key skills one needs to master to be a competent technician in the practice. Go around the room several times, writing down what people say on the whiteboard. You will probably generate a list of 30 or more discrete skills, ranging from how to escort and interact with patients to how to assist in surgery.

2. At the same meeting (or a subsequent meeting if you've run out of time) ask the techs to write a "B" for basic, "I" for intermediate, or "A" for advanced next to each skill you have written on the board.
3. Then assign each meeting participant one of the "B"-for-basic skills to write out over the next week or two in an agreed-upon word processing format (furnish a sample format of how you would like these first drafts to look).
4. The tech manager then edits the first drafts and passes these along to a designated doctor (or the entire professional staff) for approval.
5. When each set is completed, the techs are assigned the next topic from the whiteboard, moving from the basic items to the advanced ones.
6. Repeat this process every week or two until the operations manual is finished and formally approved.

In larger practices, with lots of techs, you can write the entire tech manual—50 pages or longer—in a month or two. In smaller practices, where there are fewer staff who can often be more intensely employed, with little downtime for writing protocols, it may take a year to complete a department's operations manual.

This same week-by-week process can be pursued in every department, and in a matter of a few months in most settings will result in a completed operations manual for the entire practice.

Take a look at the simple, sample protocol for performing a confrontation vision field. The art of writing a protocol is to strike a balance between too much and too little detail.

After putting in this effort, even though it was comparatively painless for you as a practice leader, you will want to use your new operations manual as a live document:

- As an orientation and training manual for new staff, and as refresher course material throughout the year for even the most senior staff
- As a tool to help with annual recredentialing of technical and other staff
- As the basis for auditing work processes and looking for greater efficiencies
- To help new doctors in the practice understand how support staff do their work
- As a living document, making additions throughout the year as new protocols come to light, and reading the manual deeply from cover-to-cover once a year, making any needed corrections or changes

Example Only

Department: Technical services

Protocol 15: Confrontation fields

Effective: October 2021

Purpose: To provide a simple screening examination of the patient's peripheral vision.

Procedure: (Always be sure to explain the procedure to the patient.)

1. Have the patient cover the left eye first and look at your nose.
2. Instruct the patient not to look at your fingers.
3. Close your right eye.
4. Holding your fingers up (superior, inferior, nasal, and temporal), have the patient look at your nose.
5. The patient should be able to count your fingers.
6. Proceed with the opposite eye.
7. If you are able to see your fingers, the patient should be able to see them as well.
8. If an area is detected of decreased vision, bring fingers inward until seen by the patient.
9. Document in the chart where the defect is located
10. If a visual field defect is noted, proceed with automated visual field.

CHAPTER 8

Checklists to Help You Stay Organized and Efficient

The obvious rule of efficiency is you don't want to spend more time organizing than it's worth.
—Daniel Levitin

Rename your "To-Do" list to your "Opportunities" list. Each day is a treasure chest filled with limitless opportunities; take joy in checking many off your list.
—Steve Maraboli

Under conditions of complexity, not only are checklists a help, they are required for success.
—Atul Gawande

The complexity of running an ophthalmic practice is underappreciated by most new arrivers to the ophthalmic workplace. Here's an example:

We received a phone call from the practice administrator of a $10 million practice in the Midwest. She had enthusiastically accepted the position 6 months before, thinking it was a great, calming career move. She had stepped away from being the CEO of a 350-bed hospital and had wanted the last few years of her career to be less demanding than running a hospital.

Wohl C, Pinto JB. *UP: Taking Ophthalmic Administrators and Their Management Teams to the Next Level of Skill, Performance, and Career Satisfaction, Second Edition* (pp 47-50).

After just 6 months on the job, she was resigning. "I had no idea it was so hard to run a simple practice like this," she said. She had misjudged the talent and knowledge needed to run an ophthalmic practice, a "surprisingly" complex organization.

If you run an ophthalmology practice, you can probably relate. There's the built-in pressure of the profession: the field of ophthalmology creates a culture of exactitude. There are layers of the organizational complexity. And, in addition to the complexity, the raw number of "customers" coming through the door each day drives such an energetic pace that it's easy to drown.

In the face of operational complexity, discipline is needed. And one of the best tools to impose this discipline is the use of checklists.

Pilots figured this out a long time ago. Even the smartest and most experienced pilot, flying the smallest plane, uses checklists to ensure that all systems are operational. The larger the plane, the longer the checklist. Checklists help you and your management team keep your practice "airborne." And there is value in having more than just one master checklist in your practice. If you are the administrator, you may have an overall checklist of big things that have to be ticked off during the course of the year, but you will also find value in monthly, weekly, even daily checklists to stay on top of the details. Each of your department heads may have their own checklists and more detailed reminder lists to be used by their rank-and-file workers.

A checklist is an accountability document that helps to create a deliberate, linear process. Checklists break down larger procedures, provide structure, and help ensure that critical steps are not missed.

• • •

Following are limited, sample departmental checklists that you can implement in your practice. Revise and expand these samples to fit the needs of each department. This is best done as a department-level brainstorming exercise. Think about how the department works on the best days and memorialize the success steps followed on such days. Then focus on any current trouble spots, and add items to the list to keep these problems from surfacing.

Your checklist should be a living document, modified over time as new challenges arise. Launching and editing this checklist over time is a wonderful way to help newer managers focus on the success factors in their department and get accustomed to the granular attention to detail obliged in an eye clinic.

Reception and Patient Accounts Department Checklist

____ The computer system has been backed up daily and the data stored off-site or in the cloud.

____ The phones have been covered satisfactorily this week.

____ Emergency patients have been worked into the schedule and seen cheerfully.

____ There is no more than a 5-day delay to the next surgical/urgent appointment slot.

_____ There is no more than a 15-day delay to the next routine appointment slot.
_____ The no-show rate this week has been at or under 5%.
_____ All no-show patients have been called within 1 hour.
_____ Primary waiting time has not exceeded 20 minutes for any doctor.
_____ New patients have been fairly distributed among the doctors this week.
_____ Patients have been notified 24 to 48 hours in advance to remind them of their appointment.
_____ Payment type and eligibility have been always verified before each exam or surgery.
_____ Front desk staff have entered accurate and complete demographic data.
_____ All possible patient-responsible amounts have been collected at the time of service.
_____ Charges have been posted within 24 hours of services being provided.
_____ Insurance claims have been submitted within 48 hours of services being provided.
_____ Payments have been posted and deposits made within 24 hours.
_____ Secondary claims have been submitted promptly.
_____ Collections work has proceeded satisfactorily this week.
_____ Delinquent patients have been turned over to a collection agency.
_____ Day-end closings have been timely and all drawers balanced.
_____ Lasers, special testing equipment logs, and retinal injection medication usage have been cross-checked against charges submitted.
_____ Third-party payments have been timely, and payments match the fee schedule in contractual agreements.
_____ Payment denials have been appealed when unreasonable.

Clinical Services Department

_____ Doctors have arrived in the clinic at least 10 minutes before their first patient is worked up.
_____ Techs, scribes, and doctors have entered accurate and complete chart and superbill data.
_____ Agreed-upon care pathways have been followed and audited.
_____ Charts have been checked randomly for missing information, missed charges, lack of continuity of care, and missed opportunities to provide needed services.
_____ Special testing ordered has been followed up.
_____ Dictation has been completed within 48 hours and consult letters sent within 1 week.
_____ All surgical patients received an evening call from their surgeon or a staff member.

Marketing and Outreach Department

_____ All departing patients have been encouraged to refer the practice.

_____ All appropriate departing patients have been either reappointed or put in the recall system.

_____ Patients who refer their friends/family have received thank you notes and calls.

_____ Referral sources have been entered in the computer.

_____ All providers (and any designated staff) are on track in reaching out to referral sources.

_____ The practice website is current and operational.

_____ The administrator and managing partner take a field trip visit together to at least one superior practice each year to get new marketing/development/patient service ideas.

_____ Total marketing outlays are a fit with new patient growth goals, neither over- nor undershooting requirements.

Other common department checklists include: human resources, office facilities management, risk management, legal affairs and regulatory compliance, and managing partner responsibilities.

As the administrator, you may receive pushback from selected managers who don't want to be held accountable or who are concerned that checklists will make them appear to be micromanaging their staff. You can provide your managers with "cover" by attending scheduled department meetings from time to time and letting staff know why attention to detail is critical. Let them know that their checklists are being imposed by you and the board, not by an overcontrolling department head. Most importantly, let line staff participate in the refinement of their checklists, so that they become their tools as much as accountability documents for practice leaders.

CHAPTER 9

Management's Role in Boosting Each Patient's Experience

Southwest Airlines is successful because the company understands it's a customer service company that just happens to be an airline.
—Harvey Mackay

Customer service is just a day-in, day-out, ongoing, never-ending, unremitting, persevering, compassionate type of activity.
—Leon Gorman

Few patients have a background allowing them to gauge the objective quality of the eye care they receive. But every one of your patients is a perfect instrument when it comes to measuring the caring and value they receive from your practice. They know "20/happy" when they get it at your practice.

Although doctors are at the heart of providing ophthalmic care, your management team is the front line for ensuring a high level of customer satisfaction.

Here's a quick assessment you can take to determine how you and your managers—and the overall practice enterprise—are doing in fostering patient contentment. Following are 20 activities and attributes that help to drive higher levels of patient satisfaction. Rank each on a 0 to 5 scale (where "0" means your practice does this very poorly or not at all and "5" means your practice excels at this).

Wohl C, Pinto JB. *UP: Taking Ophthalmic Administrators and Their Management Teams to the Next Level of Skill, Performance, and Career Satisfaction, Second Edition* (pp 51-54).

_____ 1. We have formally designated a member of our practice to be in charge of monitoring and improving each patient's experience during his or her visit with our practice. (This can be the administrator, a department head, or a provider.)

_____ 2. We have agreed on and written out the hallmarks of what we think it means to deliver an excellent experience for patients, including such things as maximum waiting and total visit time, addressing each patient's chief complaint specifically, making sure the patient leaves knowing what he or she should do next about any medical condition, etc.

_____ 3. In our practice, we consider a complaining patient an early warning sign of something we could be doing better, because we know that for every patient who complains about something there are probably many who suffer in silence.

_____ 4. We have a formal, written process for logging and responding to patient complaints. Once a problem has been logged, a manager or the practice administrator has to close the case formally and sign off that the patient's concerns have been appropriately addressed.

_____ 5. Our practice has training materials for teaching both staff and providers how to provide a more caring, patient-friendly environment and how to respond to everything from minor grumbles to major service mishaps.

_____ 6. Our administrator and mid-level managers receive ongoing, specific training not only on customer care but on how to train staff on the elements of providing superior customer service as well. We train the trainers so that our customer service mission is constantly improving for the better.

_____ 7. During staff meetings, we often bring up examples of good and poor customer service, so that our team develops widely understood standards for patient care and caring over time.

_____ 8. At the time of our annual staff and doctor performance reviews, each member of our practice is graded on, among other things, their sensitivity to and success at providing each patient with a great experience in our practice. If the performance score is low, we initiate remedial training and subsequent oversight.

_____ 9. We manage patient expectations so that they match what we can reasonably deliver. An example would be to tell a patient at check-in if the practice is running on time, or advising a new surgical consult patient that their appointment will involve extra testing that will be more time consuming.

_____ 10. During the course of a patient's visit to our office, we ask a lot of checking in questions: "Do you have any special needs or questions during today's visit?" "Are you comfortable?" "Do you have any questions about what I have just described?" "Before we wrap up today, do you have any final questions for me?"

_____ 11. Because we know it is sometimes uncomfortable to have an eye exam, and some patients are especially apprehensive, we work hard to comfort and soothe anxieties. We do this by adjusting our tone of voice, not rushing, and letting patients know ahead of time when something uncomfortable (eg, a bright light, needle stick) is about to happen.

_____ 12. We formally measure and report on patient satisfaction. (There are numerous ways to do this: written surveys, phone surveys, focus groups.) We track our progress over time, and have agreed on an objective, minimum score that we work to exceed consistently.

_____ 13. Our administrator routinely gets up and walks the clinic floor, first to observe directly and ensure that the practice is running smoothly and second to engage patients in a friendly conversation about how their visit is going. An example (spoken to a patient in the sub-waiting/dilating areas) is: "Hi, I'm Anita, the practice's administrator. How are we doing for you today? Is there anything we could improve today or on future visits?"

_____ 14. The first staff that most patients meet are our phone operators and receptionists. Because these workers set the tone for how the rest of the visit will go, we hire and train for exceptional warmth and friendliness in these roles. We only pick staff who can be cheerful to the grumpiest people over and over again throughout the day.

_____ 15. Because patients spend more time with technical staff than with any other workers in the practice, the head technician is our most vigilant customer satisfaction monitor. He or she questions techs and scribes closely for any evidence of service gaps, adverse patient–doctor interaction, a lack of gentle treatment or a kind word.

_____ 16. We know that for most patients, their chief complaint in the clinic is not "dry eye" or "blurry vision" but "excess waiting time." Accordingly, managers in each department conduct regular time studies and have not-to-exceed standards their teams need to hit.

_____ 17. We observe the basics of being a good host to our visitors: a scrupulously clean facility, enough space and seating so that everyone is comfortably accommodated, access for patients with disabilities, refreshments, calming background music, and interesting reading material to help pass the time.

_____ 18. In addition to paying attention to complaints, we listen carefully to patient compliments, and use these to better understand what patients like and how we can deliver more of that.

_____ 19. One of the most important traits we look for when hiring new staff and doctors is their friendliness and empathy for the feelings of our patients. We can teach anyone how to answer the phone or run a visual field test, but it's hard to teach someone how to like people and serve them in a manner that leaves them delighted with the care they received.

_____ 20. We briskly remove or reassign staff who are not patient-friendly. In addition to knowing how to perform the technical components of their job consistently, every staff member needs to know how to delight patients. We have dismissed staff who complete their core job functions well but didn't meet our standards of customer care.

The maximum potential score on this is 100 points. Add up your practice's score. Note any especially weak areas for priority attention. Hold a group discussion with your management team.

Remember that a patient's level of satisfaction is simply the comparison between expectations and experience. In all service sectors, customer expectations are rising, at the same time that your patients have the ability to very publicly score their perception of the service you provide. In addition, third-party payers commonly make their panel decisions as much on patient complaints as they do on adverse utilization or outcomes. In an increasingly transparent and judgmental world, managers are as much a determinant of practice success as the surgeons they serve.

Section II

Boosting Career Consciousness and Effectiveness

CHAPTER 10

Are You Pursuing an Intentional or an Accidental Career?

The driving force of a career must come from the individual. Remember: Jobs are owned by the company, you own your career!
—Earl Nightingale

My career is a journey for me, and any journey is incomplete without the struggle
—Yami Gautam

Having spoken with a few thousand ophthalmic administrators and senior department heads in the last 40+ years, we can report that many business careers in eye care are at least partially accidental. Happy accidents, to be sure, but certainly not the result of much intentional planning. We'd like to change that with what follows.

Ask yourself this simple question: On a 0 to 10 scale, how diligently and energetically do you work for the doctors who own your practice? For your staff? Your patients? Now ask a parallel question on the same 0 to 10 scale: How diligently and energetically do you work to develop your professional career?

If you are like most of your peers, your score for the first question is a lot higher than for the second question. If you're in your office as you're reading this,

Wohl C, Pinto JB. *UP: Taking Ophthalmic Administrators and Their Management Teams to the Next Level of Skill, Performance, and Career Satisfaction, Second Edition* (pp 57-60).

look around. You have books, papers, and e-files aplenty related to managing your practice. But probably precious little related to managing the next 5 or 10 or 30 years of your career.

This runs against the modern understanding of how to be an enlightened professional in the 21st century. No matter how kind, loyal, embracing, and supportive your board is, no matter how much you love your job and want to stay there forever, odds are you will have at least two or three more positions before your career winds down.

That's why your peers in other industries increasingly see themselves in two jobs simultaneously: Their current, orthodox job title (something like "VP of Operations") and their less obvious but equally important job title as "CEO of Me, Inc."

Let's explore what's involved for you to be an effective CEO of Me, Inc—what it takes to manage your career as intentionally as you manage your practice.

1. The starting point is to recognize that the professional scope of ophthalmic practice management has been growing vigorously over the last 20 years. The opportunities, pay scale, and prestige—along with the stress, accountability, and time commitment—have all soared. The average practice is larger, more diverse, and under more unrelenting pressure. Only by personally growing at a pace proportionate or better to the challenges faced by your current practice (much less the practice you would like to lead in the future) will your career be on a positive trajectory. Ask yourself, "Am I personally ahead or behind this growth curve?" (By the way, this is the same line of questioning the most thoughtful surgeons we all work for ask themselves often and struggle with in their own way to keep up with a fast-moving professional domain.)
2. Next, recognize and prepare for the greatest industry trends coming over the horizon for all health care executives, especially if you are a younger administrator or department head:
    - The historically dominant small/private practice model for ophthalmology will increasingly yield to three leading models: The large private practice (through merger-consolidation), the aggregation of small practices into supergroups under private equity models, and consolidations under regional health systems. These larger, more corporate enterprises oblige a more professionalized executive cohort, with more formal training and a much higher level of accountability to the bottom line.
    - Practice profit margins are generally falling, so financial sophistication is an essential job skill; you don't have to become a CPA, but your bookkeeping and financial analysis skills, at the very least, must edge up a notch.
    - Regulatory burdens are rising so every administrator is increasingly in a guardian role, working with outside specialists to stay on the correct side of a very punishing line.

3. As the CEO of Me, Inc, your chief job (like every other CEO) is to boost shareholder value and enterprise sustainability. What does this mean to you as Me, Inc's leader? It means more than just being technically excellent at the nitty gritty details of your job. It means you also must work daily on your *brand equity*, which is just a fancy term for your reputation as a leader. Ask yourself: Compared to a year ago, is my reputation in my current practice—the admiration that people here have for the work I do—higher or lower today? You can also ask, if you are thinking a few steps ahead in your career, "What's my reputation in the national community?" If you are destined to achieve higher executive levels, leading larger practices or even consulting, now is the time to write articles, give talks and broaden your network of industry contacts.
4. You should have a written, personal career plan, analogous to your practice's strategic business plan. A reasonable planning horizon for a mid-career practice administrator is at least 10 years, and your plan should answer questions like these:
   - How high is up? What will my dream job be at the apex of my career?
   - What is my planning horizon? How many more years do I have to not only achieve my dream job, but also stay with it long enough to leave a lasting legacy?
   - What do I need to learn to get my dream job? Where can I learn this? Just reading and visiting peers in other practices and going to national conferences? Or do I need to go back to school? Will my current practice or my next practice help support my education?
   - What other resources do I need? Money for continuing education? Support from my spouse? More stamina for the high stress and long hours ahead?
   - Am I willing to pay the toll: Time, family sacrifices, the inevitable risk every time I try out a new position?
   - If on reflection my career goals are more modest (and that's fine, too) or I am already working in my dream job, I probably still need to keep tuning up my skills. What would that look like?
5. If income is important to you, realize that the wage you earn in medical management generally depends on the scale of practice you lead. You may be running a $2 million practice with two doctors seeing 10,000 patient visits per year today, with a typical base salary of $90,000. Want more? With the right planning and preparation, and a bit of good fortune, you could lead a $20 million practice serving 50,000 patients per year, with a base salary of $250,000. The leap from the first practice to the second, larger one is unlikely to be accomplished overnight in one job change. But a couple of smaller hops taken over 5 to 10 years can result in this level of financial promotion.
6. Perhaps more importantly, for those who consider their job in health care to be a kind of public service, a calling, the influence you ultimately have on great patient care will depend on how far your career goes. Many practice administrators and department heads grew up wanting to be doctors or nurses. The truth? As an executive in a larger medical practice, odds are high that you are in a better position to influence public health than you ever would have achieved as a direct provider of patient care.

7. Finally, recognize that every development effort—whether corporately for your practice or personally for your career—requires risk, effort, and a commitment of time. The competent CEO of a $20 million practice needs to work 50+ hours a week. And there is a proportionately greater employment tenure risk when you rise to higher career levels. Keeping two doctors happy in a modest practice is a lot easier than keeping a board of 10 doctors happy. And if you should lose your job as the CEO of a $20 million ophthalmic practice, it is going to take much longer to find an equivalent position compared to losing your job as administrator of a $2 million practice. And you'll likely have to relocate.

Consider all your options, including the exciting new professional options emerging as practice scale is growing. Be conscious. Be intentional. Choose wisely. Work hard. Most importantly, thrive ... no matter what kind of career you create.

CHAPTER 11

What's the Difference Between an Office Manager and an Administrator?

A leader is someone who knows the way,
goes the way, and shows the way.
—John C. Maxwell

Management is doing things right;
leadership is doing the right things.
—Peter Drucker

About 10 times per week we say to physician clients: "If you want to be a great business owner, don't try to think like a business person, think like a doctor. Think of your practice's benchmarks and financial statements as a kind of lab report. Practices can grow cold or run a fever, just like a human patient."

The same nexus between business and medicine can be applied to the often-confused difference and blurred lines between an office manager and an administrator (or otherwise-elevated provider of practice oversight: executive director or even CEO in the largest settings). Here's how:

Wohl C, Pinto JB. *UP: Taking Ophthalmic Administrators and Their Management Teams to the Next Level of Skill, Performance, and Career Satisfaction, Second Edition* (pp 61-64).

- Office managers are generally like an ophthalmic technician. With supervision they can (largely by rote) gather practice data, check on staffer performance, and report to the higher-ups. They can't take action without specific orders.
- Administrators are generally like a physician. An MD, DO, or OD has training that allows them to do a technician's basic work-up, and then go beyond this to gather more invasive data, frame a diagnosis, and commence a treatment plan. Physicians are licensed to provide the full arc of care, whereas techs must stop short at gathering the basic patient information and running a few simple tests.

Which one are you? An office managing "tech" or an administrating "doctor?" How do you know?

We're not making a value judgment here, the world needs both junior and senior business types, just as it needs junior and senior caregivers. Obviously one is not better than the other. They each have their own roles, duties, authorities, and limits.

To help you understand what side of the line you are on (and perhaps encourage you to step up to the next level in your career) here are nine dimensions of the administrator vs office manager dichotomy.

#1. Education

Educational achievement can be a weak gauge of an administrator's or office manager's fitness to serve. We've seen high school drop-outs run splendid practices, and MBAs blow practices apart. However, generally speaking, administrators—at least the youngest ones today—are more formally educated than office managers.

#2. Experience

Experience is a much more useful proxy for management skill in an ambulatory health care setting. Business management theory can, of course, be absorbed in a classroom, but business is not one of the so-called learned professions, in the way that medicine, law, and engineering are. The best practice executives we know are a repository of business case histories, the good, bad, and ugly, gained over decades of experience. Administrators have grayer hair than office managers.

#3. Numeracy

Two generations ago, you could be a great practice manager by knowing how to take care of patients or how to market or how to provide great customer service. You didn't have to possess a head for figures and a love of math. That has all changed today. The most important business competency separating administrators from office managers today is numeracy. Numbers allow you to diagnose and treat practice problems while they are still small. Numbers allow you to hold people more accountable for their performance. Numbers allow you to better communicate goals.

#4. Responsibility

Just as doctors, not techs, are ultimately accountable for patient outcomes, administrators have a comparable life-or-death accountability for the health of their "patients." Office managers rarely have a profit and loss responsibility—they more often have a *process responsibility*. They are more responsible for smooth, rather than profitable, operations.

#5. Resource Allocation Authority

An administrator translates the board's mandate into an action plan and is granted the necessary and enduring (often growing) authority to carry out that plan. Office managers often have to take baby steps, going back and forth to the doctor or board for incremental permission to take the next step.

#6. Independence

Administrators (like doctors) don't have to check in all the time with a higher authority. They can make a wide range of independent decisions. Office managers play an extended game of adult "Father/Mother, May I?," checking in often for approval on even trivial decisions.

#7. Relationships With Practice Owners

The best ophthalmic practices in the United States are co-run by a strong doctor-leader working in lockstep with a strong administrative leader. Administrators should feel like, and be treated like, near-peers of practice owners. This should have a nearly co-parenting feeling, where "mom and dad" stand as a strong and united front, to raise the "kids" with an equal measure of kindness and firmness. Most office managers are relegated in most cases to being minions, definitely not on the same intellectual or career commitment level as the providers, at least in the provider's mind.

#8. Strategic Intimacy

Administrators are generally on the inside track of where the practice is heading in the future, at least to the extent that the owners are themselves thinking about the big picture. Office managers, on the other hand, live a kind of *Groundhog Day* life, named after the film where the lead, played by Bill Murray, lives the same day over and over again. Managers generally have a short planning horizon and are not used by their doctors as sounding boards for future planning.

#9. Leadership

Much has been written about the difference between managing and leading. One of John's SLACK books, *Ophthalmic Leadership: A Practical Guide for Physicians, Administrators, and Teams, Second Edition*, is devoted to the subject. Generally, administrators can both manage and lead their organizations. They carry themselves and relate to others in a manner eliciting respect, trust, and a desire to follow. While many office managers working in practices today may one day become very good leaders, they are at present staff sergeants at best, and have not yet risen up the ranks.

• • •

Of course, all things are relative. Some doctors give their lead lay staffer the junior title of office manager, but give them more authority than the CEOs of some practices. And vice versa.

If you're called an administrator but are really only granted limited authority, you may want to share this article with your board and ask for a longer leash. If you are presently an office manager and are ready to spread your wings, talk to your employer about training and development work that can help take you to the next level of your career. And use the tools and guidance within this book to step up to the next level of your career.

CHAPTER 12

The Value of a Mentor at Every Stage of Your Career

What I need is someone who will make me do what I can.
—Ralph Waldo Emerson

If you want happiness for a lifetime—help others.
—Chinese proverb

The delicate balance of mentoring someone is not creating them in your own image, but giving them the opportunity to create themselves.
—Steven Spielberg

There are many differences between good and great administrators. Great administrators possess more curiosity, more discipline, and more perseverance. Great administrators achieve a higher level of technical mastery; they hate being in the dark. They are more obsessive about the details. They place high value on continuing education for themselves and others.

Great administrators carry themselves with a confidence borne of lots of career wins, which reinforces their leadership chops in the boardroom and allows them to get faster approval, leading to even more accomplishments … a virtuous cycle.

Wohl C, Pinto JB. *UP: Taking Ophthalmic Administrators and Their Management Teams to the Next Level of Skill, Performance, and Career Satisfaction, Second Edition* (pp 65-67).

How do most great administrators become great? Formal education is a start, but only a start. The most prominent factor can be summed up on one word: Mentoring (which is actually a very specialized form of education, and a subset of the lifelong learning movement).

Mentoring falls halfway between a traditional educational relationship, like being back in college, and (in the very best of mentoring relationships) the kind of nonjudgmental, affirming support that effective parents provide.

Mentoring is kindly, generous, and forgiving, quite different from the stern expectations of a boss or high school teacher.

As an administrator (or department head or physician) reading this book, you should be sensitive to the value of education … not just in the formal schooling sense, but in the day-to-day sense. A former biochemistry professor of John's once said, "Life is nothing more than teaching and learning." If you think about it, that's what you are doing all week long.

1. You get the most recent aging report.
2. You learn from the data that open accounts are growing stale.
3. You meet with your billing supervisor and collaboratively learn about a payer slowdown and understaffing in the department.
4. Then you teach the billing department how to resolve the acute cash flow pinch, and teach your board about your findings, missing resources, and the action plan to implement.

•••

As the demands of managing an ophthalmology practice have grown exponentially, where expectations are high and the pace is faster each year, mentees absolutely appreciate the assistance of their mentors. But the gift of mentoring goes both ways. If you're old enough and have enough experience, being a mentor is one the greatest professional gifts you can give … to yourself.

All too often new administrators are isolated from peers. With a nose to the grindstone and few local administrators who are not competitors, it's easy to see how this happens. Even those of you who travel to national meetings may be challenged to pick one mentor out of the hundreds potentially available in the hallways.

Speaking from personal experience, I (Corinne) have had several mentors over a span of more than 30 years in hospital and physician practice administration. The career stage I was in at the time dictated who was most valuable to me. As a new graduate, I was a sponge for everything my early mentors shared. Thirty years on, I'm still blotting up pearls, both from my formal mentors and informally from a cross-section of business colleagues in and out of medicine.

As an experienced professional coach and mentor, I can share that often the mentee already has good instincts and core theoretical knowledge. What the mentee needs most is case histories, examples of what works on the street, things that will reinforce book learning. And most of all, the mentee needs positive feedback and encouragement.

What mentors provide is not the same thing found in a business journal or grad school lecture. Often it has to do with relationship building or critical and strategic thinking and how to work better with physicians. And it's interesting to realize when you talk to someone who has less experience than you, you gain an appreciation for the skills you have attained over the years.

To get the most value out of your mentor, set a monthly or bimonthly appointment (in person or over the phone) and be prepared with questions or situations to share. Jot these down throughout the month, and the list will be ready for your meeting. You will find that time spent together quickly turns into a mutual sharing and both parties always learn something … it is impossible to teach without learning yourself. If your mentor is a fellow administrator, arrange to visit his or her practice, bring your managers with you, and learn how your mentor runs a practice from many different perspectives.

Finding a mentor, this special kind of teacher in your life, is easy, though many hold back from seeking one. The presumption among young executives is that older colleagues couldn't be bothered aiding a junior manager. Don't be shy. Mentors get as much out of the experience as mentees.

Being an effective mentee is also easy. There are just five rules:

1. Match your unique needs with a mentor's unique abilities. You may be lucky enough to find an all-purpose mentor, but there is no rule saying you can only have one mentor at a time. Have your CPA mentor you on financial analysis while your favorite doctor in the practice mentors you on the medical science of ophthalmology.
2. You are responsible for starting the relationship. It is as simple as saying: "I really admire how you _____________. I would like to get better at that. Would you consider being my mentor in this area?"
3. You are responsible for fostering the relationship. Like friendships, mentor–mentee relationships need feeding. Stay in touch (but not to the point of pestering). Try everything your mentor suggests (don't be resistant or noncompliant). Give feedback on how your mentor's ideas are working out.
4. Don't waste your mentor's time. Prepare for each mentoring session. Ask intelligent questions that only your mentor can answer, not something you could have looked up online.
5. Show gratitude. Give something back to your mentor. Let him or her learn specifically about your progress. Even after the formal mentoring relationship ends, send a letter or email from time to time about how you are still progressing because of the jump start your mentor so generously furnished.

Giving is always more satisfying then receiving, and at this stage in both our careers, this is one way we give back for what we received. Most experienced administrators feel the same way. So we encourage you to reach out and find a mentor. It truly is a gift for both sides.

CHAPTER 13

Coaching Up and Down the Ranks to Enhance Practice Performance

Really, coaching is simplicity. It's getting players to play better than they think that they can.
—Tom Landry

I hired top-notch people, trusted then to do their jobs, and then came to grips with the fact that I wouldn't be coaching as much.
—Tony Dungy

Horace Greeley, famous in the 1800s for saying, "Go west, young man," was a hard-working, rags-to-riches statesman and publisher who also said, "Common sense is very uncommon." There is nothing more uncommon in the business of ophthalmology than the recognition that your practice is the sum of its parts—each of which must be groomed individually if you hope to provide superior patient care.

This doesn't just mean cultivating your tangible office facilities, testing equipment, and website. As important as these are, they only represent about 30% of the typical practice's operational outlay and an even smaller portion of your success as an ophthalmic enterprise.

Wohl C, Pinto JB. *UP: Taking Ophthalmic Administrators and Their Management Teams to the Next Level of Skill, Performance, and Career Satisfaction, Second Edition* (pp 69-72).

More crucially, you chiefly have to improve the most expensive and delicate part of your practice: your people. Doctor and lay staff wages make up 70% of the typical practice's cash flow, but a much larger portion of your success.

Your practice, at its root, is a team of people where numerous individual doctor, manager, and line staff careers are continuously offered up to be groomed (and not infrequently repaired) by you as a leader.

As an administrator, managing partner, or department head in your practice, if you can improve the performance of each of these distinct individual teammates, the entire practice team improves. So, let's substitute the word "coaching" here for "managing," because the continuous improvement of human performance is central to ophthalmic business management. You may manage inventories. Or vendors. Or facilities. But you need to *coach* people.

What Is Coaching?

Whether you are coaching your employees or doctors, several generic principles of effective coaching apply. These principles are the same in business and medicine as in athletics. Let's explore some of these.

First, as a coach in your practice, you need to understand baseline performance. In baseball, basketball, and football, the coaching staff have a working knowledge of the optimal performance to be expected in their respective sports. The very best players may be able to approach a 0.3 batting average, or 20 points in a basketball game, or a 50% pass completion ratio in football.

As an ophthalmology coach you need to know what great performance looks like. For example, you should know that a technician should be able to work up the average new patient in less than 20 minutes. Or that a phone operator can easily handle 15 calls in an hour. Or that a motivated general ophthalmologist can readily see more than 20 patient encounters in a morning.

Although ophthalmology is hardly as competitive as the Super Bowl, you still need to know what *winning* means. This is easy in football. The team with the most points wins. How about in ophthalmology? Winning is a bit more diffuse and includes:

- Patients being served pleasantly and on time
- Each patient's chief complaints being addressed
- Treatment outcomes that equal or exceed contemporary professional standards
- Referring doctors getting needed feedback on the status of their patients
- Providers and staff enjoying their day and earning a fair wage

If you are not counting up your points in each of these dimensions, how do you know it's been a great month? If you've won the Super Bowl? Not only do you personally need to know how to read the scoreboard, but staff and doctors need to all agree on what constitutes a winning score. Post the key practice stats (eg, monthly visits, cases, no-show rates) in the break room. Be sure to cover key performance indicators (eg, financial statements, cash position, surgical density, average collections per visit) in monthly board meetings.

When you win, everyone should be included in the celebration. Does your practice call out its winning players and team wins? If not, start now with staff citations, bonuses, and awards for most-improved player. As important as celebrating wins, when you lose the game because of poor profits, disgruntled patients, or a clinic that runs behind, gather the involved players. Determine why you lost. What drove disappointing profits this quarter:

- Competition?
- Undue provider time away from the practice?
- Lags in the billing department?
- Unplanned expenses?

Great ophthalmic coaches realize that while most players are committed and eager to play hard, a few of your team members may not really be engaged. You may need to cut the players who should not be on your team or you find resistant and uncoachable.

As the administrator, managing doctor, or department head, the most important person you must learn to coach is yourself. Recognizing what does and does not motivate you is an excellent step toward understanding how coaching can impact others. This may sound like an extremely simple idea, but you might be surprised how many managers, in a very busy practice environment, manage "from the hip" without putting a lot of thought into process and outcomes.

Take the time to make your coaching approach intentionally. The brief self-test that follows will help you score how well you're doing as the coach of your practice.

A Practice Leader's Coaching Test

Mark the following 15 items on a 0 to 3 score.

0 = Never

1 = Occasionally

2 = Frequently

3 = Always

When you finish, select three items at which you are weakest, and write down a brief improvement plan. Share your results with whomever you report to: the board if you are the managing partner, the managing partner if you are the administrator, or the administrator if you are a department head. Then review your score and your improvement plan quarterly to check for progress or regression.

____ 1. I readily accept constructive, even negative feedback, from my team members.

____ 2. When meeting with my team, I listen more than half of the time.

____ 3. I assume that everyone on the team has hidden talents that I just have not been able to bring out yet.

____ 4. While always willing to make suggestions, I try first to help my players find their own solutions to their problems.

____ 5. My coaching style is to catch my players doing things right, and encouraging more, rather than pointing out what's been done wrong.

_____ 6. I am unafraid of confrontation when it is necessary to correct poor performance.

_____ 7. I am as comfortable confronting subordinate staff about difficult issues as I am confronting peers and my superiors.

_____ 8. Before trying to coach a player, I first make sure that I understand their motivations and goals.

_____ 9. My style is most often suggestive, rather than directive, when I coach.

_____ 10. When I listen to a player, I also watch for nonverbal clues.

_____ 11. Before describing a desired new performance goal with a player, I make sure that we both agree on the strengths and weaknesses of their past performance.

_____ 12. After I've discussed a desired new performance standard with a player, I make sure they understand what's in it for them if they are able to reach this new standard.

_____ 13. At the end of a "coaching moment" with one of my staff or doctors, I make sure I have their commitment. When appropriate, we put things in writing and even have players sign off their commitment formally.

_____ 14. I make notes about the work that I do with my players, so I can refer back to our progress and we can all remember what the goals were.

_____ 15. Knowing that I can't coach alone, when appropriate I enlist the help of other co-coaches, including other staff and doctors, outside advisors, a doctor's spouse, etc.

CHAPTER 14

Wohl's Administrator Success Factors

Success means doing the best we can with what we have. Success is the doing, not the getting; in the trying, not the triumph. Success is a personal standard, reaching for the highest that is in us, becoming all that we can be.
—Zig Ziglar

Wise leaders set personal standards of excellence. Top performers focus on looking forward, despite what happened in the past.

If we placed you and other accomplished administrators in a room and asked each of you to list the main success factors of your career, it's likely the following 12 items would percolate to the top of the list.

I've sat exactly where you now sit for more than a third of my career. I've lived your same practice management challenges daily, and know that while we could easily create a longer list of success factors, nailing these 12 can lead the way to creating a more successful and satisfying career.

Add these 12 success factors to your personal framework for success. Replace good intentions with earned results. Stay on the course you set for yourself and your team. Winning standards like these will take you, your career, and your practice far ahead in the years ahead.

Wohl's Administrator Success Factors

1. Be energetic at all times. Energy is contagious. Pass it on.
2. Be decisive. Don't let perfectionism slow you down or allow you to get stuck.
3. Be accountable, which is the only way you can hold others accountable.
4. Business is like a diet. The intent to change is meaningless. Action alone has value.
5. At every moment in your career, you should have a mentor and be a mentor.
6. You can best improve things you can measure. Make all your decisions data-driven.
7. Be aligned with your board. Communicate and execute its directives clearly.
8. Inspire mostly by helping people feel better about themselves.
9. Ask the question "Why?" more often. Find and treat the root of every problem.
10. Change is the one constant. Don't resist change. Make it a friend.
11. Be trustworthy and honest, even at the risk of adverse personal consequences.
12. Work harder than everyone else. Limitations are more self-imposed than real. Stretch.

Section III

Mid-Level Manager Development

CHAPTER 15

Strong Department Leaders Make Strong Practices

The way management treats associates is exactly how the associates will treat the customers.
—Sam Walton

Leaders are made, they are not born. They are made by hard effort, which is the price which all of us must pay to achieve any goal that is worthwhile.
—Vince Lombardi

If you are working in a large practice as the administrator, you already know that your middle managers can make or break you. They will either act as a flawless support team that handles the bulk of day-to-day operations, freeing up time for the administrator to focus on higher-level responsibilities like strategic planning. Or your middle managers will require constant oversight and be a barrier to the growth of the practice … and your growth as the practice's leader.

Middle managers, in practices large and small, commonly play an important dual role. They act both as front-line workers and as working supervisors. This role is extremely challenging because of the cat-like balance required. Being the lead receptionist may require 20 hours per week of direct supervisory time, but with the demands of a busy office, this time block is often slivered up into an hour here or there.

Wohl C, Pinto JB. *UP: Taking Ophthalmic Administrators and Their Management Teams to the Next Level of Skill, Performance, and Career Satisfaction, Second Edition* (pp 77-83). © 2021 Taylor & Francis Group.

Being a middle manager is exhausting, and the smaller the office, the more tiresome it gets. Middle managers might as well be called that because they are inserted into the *middle* of complicated relationships with their administrator, the owners, employees, doctors, patients, and their direct staff reports. One minute they are following the leader, and a minute later they are expected to be the leader.

As an administrator, you will strengthen the core of your practice by nurturing your mid-level managers' growth in these ways:

- Provide opportunities for professional education
- Mentor actively
- Network managers to colleague-peers doing the same job in noncompeting regional practices
- Introduce them to practice management concepts that are important to you but are not yet on their radar

One of the roles of top-level practice leadership is to extract maximal value from each employee in the practice. Doing this is not just a matter of stern looks and a bossy personality, but rather of inspiring your mid-level managers to continuously look for ways of helping every staffer they supervise give more to the company.

Here is a list of skills that the best mid-level managers possess. We've included practical ideas under each category that you can expand upon as you apply these in your own practice.

Understand Management and Business Concepts

Engage your managers in areas outside their own departments by discussing how your practice works. What drives revenue production? Cost containment? Motivate and inspire by asking for their input and sharing your strategic thinking and overall practice goals. Pass down the business concepts and management tools that you have learned throughout your own career.

Human Resources Management

Human resources management is a large part of every manager's responsibility. At minimum, mid-level managers need to know how to legally interview, hire, and orient staff and how to apply a fair disciplinary process. They also need to know how to motivate staff in a professional, kindly manner, while also expecting high performance from each employee.

Conflict Resolution

This is a key skill for managers. Knowing how to stay calm, gather all the facts before leaping to conclusions, apply policies consistently, and follow up in a timely manner, especially in uncomfortable situations, is critical. Educating managers, using case histories from past errors the practice has made, is effective and reinforces the hardest lessons you have learned as a senior manager.

Numeracy: Understanding the Drivers of Economic Performance

Lots of managers brought up through the ranks fear numbers. It is common to hear "I hate numbers" and "I'm not a numbers person." There is no magic to it because few business calculations rise above sixth grade math. Teach your people how to measure practice progress through financial performance in the same way that doctors use basic testing and lab data to treat patients. Middle managers can gain this experience by having budget and key performance indicator responsibility for their own department. For example, a technical services department director should know things such as the practice's growth rate, its surgical density, and how its special testing utilization compares with peers. Such a director especially needs to understand labor productivity values like the number of tech payroll hours per patient visit.

Communication Skills

Written and oral communication skills are necessary for mid-level managers to be able to pass your message forward with clarity to their people. If your managers are not already proficient at this, you may need to employ remedial training (eg, how to write a memo or how to present effectively at a staff meeting).

Effective Delegation

Less experienced managers often believe they are better off doing a task themselves than taking the time to train others. This is a shortsighted viewpoint, but something that even some experienced managers often find difficult to grasp or feel comfortable doing. Encourage your managers to invest the time to help their own staff grow. The time taken to do so now will free up supervisory time in the future.

Organizational Skills

If you were not born an organizational wizard, you can be taught. Mid-level managers, especially working supervisors, must develop this skill to survive. Test this with questions like, "How are you preparing for the new doctor to join our practice?" If your clinic manager pulls out a two-page list she prepared, you have a great starting point. If she starts rattling off a scattered list of to-do items, she needs help.

Spend Time on the Right Things, As Prioritized by the Practice's Strategic Objectives

This is another challenging skill for new managers. Over a career, we learn how to prioritize and not let the smaller, easier projects jump in front of the larger, more important ones. We also learn to balance competing tasks. This is especially hard to do when others are pressuring you to do what is important to them at that time. Spend time with your mid-level manager reviewing prioritization skills and how to realistically determine how long each project will likely take.

Written Operational Guidelines for Each Department

Every department needs an operations manual memorializing the "one, agreed-upon, best" way to do everything. It forces service consistency, reduces errors and costs, formalizes employee training, and advances quality improvement. Make this a priority for each department manager.

Be Action-Oriented; Follow-Through and Be Accountable

There is a difference between being busy and taking effective, appropriate action. Be sure your middle managers know the difference. Hold them accountable for taking action that advances the interests of your practice. Express this expectation to them and follow up consistently, and your managers will grow.

Customer Service Focus

Medical practices, like other kinds of businesses, are being held to higher standards. Your customer service reputation is derived mainly from your front-line staff. Be sure the managers are setting high standards and leading by example.

Don't Hold Grudges. Understand the Value of Forgiveness. Staff Will Make Errors. Correct Them and Move Forward.

Managers must keep the practice moving forward. Encourage them to learn from mistakes made and to be kind to their staff, while at the same time holding each employee accountable. Teach your mid-level managers to focus more on repetitive errors that need correcting rather than the one-off human errors that happen. Newer managers have the tendency to get stuck with challenging employees and may need extra coaching in these cases. Teach the oldest truism of management: "Half of your time is spent praising your strong people and half of your time is spent replacing your weak people."

Move From Peer to Supervisor With Strength

Most mid-level managers move up through the ranks. Changing from peer to boss is not easy. All new, up-through-the-ranks managers need support in this area. Provide this assistance when a new mid-level manager is first elevated, not months later when role conflicts are starting to break down a department's function.

Turn Management Skills Into Leadership Skills

Prepare a manager development plan for each manager. (See Chapter 16 for the sample form.) Individualizing the plan to each manager's strengths, weaknesses, and career stage will help them grow as managers at their own pace. This will be more effective than the more common whole team being mentored on the same topic during a typical managers' meeting. Review the development plan with each manager quarterly and update the goals annually. You can also focus your effort to boost the team's management skills where it will best benefit the practice. Building alignment here with the practice's goals is a win for you, the managers, and the practice.

• • •

It takes tremendous self-discipline to coach yourself, let alone others. But we all do more and better with the influence of someone else pushing us to the next level. By helping your management team improve as individuals, your practice will be on the path to achieving more, too.

A Mid-Level Manager Scorecard

A list of 20 important skills possessed by some of the best mid-level department and office managers we know follows. This list is by no means complete, and no office manager could be expected to have top scores on all of these attributes. Score the most appropriate number for each item and add up the total. The maximum score is 100 points.

A Mid-Level Manager Scorecard

Score each item on a scale of 1 to 5; 1 means "I have a lot of work to do"; 3 means "I possess this skill and there is room for improvement"; and 5 reflects absolute expertise.

	Score (1 to 5)
1. Effective steward of practice resources (facility, staff, ordering)	
2. Delegation skills	
3. Human resource management	
4. Communication skills (written, oral, listening)	
5. Adaptable and flexible in the role of manager	
6. Knows how to run an effective meeting	
7. Sets the tone in the office for effective leadership	
8. Moving from peer to supervisor	
9. Works successfully with the managing partner (meetings, agenda preparation)	
10. The importance of follow-through	

(continued)

	Score (1 to 5)
11. Use of the action grid/accountability document	
12. Organizational skills (specifically applying structure to process and function)	
13. Time management skills	
14. Prioritization skills	
15. Understands key performance indicators and benchmarking	
16. Makes or contributes to data-driven decision making	
17. Knows what I don't know and seeks assistance	
18. Utilizes business-based problem-solving processes	
19. Understands regulatory demands and the resources needed	
20. Especially important to our practice is ____________________	
Total Score:	

Add up your score. With 20 different attributes, and with up to 5 points each, there's a maximum score of 100. There is no objective scale that compares you to others, but this summary score can be a valuable personal baseline of your fitness and can help point out areas to improve.

CHAPTER 16

For Administrators

Working With Each Mid-Level Manager to Create a Personalized Career Development Plan

Champions keep playing until they get it right.
—Billie Jean King

Individual commitment to a group effort—that is what makes a team work, a company work, a society work, a civilization work.
—Vince Lombardi

Being a middle manager is exhausting. Department heads are at the center of complex, high-pressure relationships, squeezed by leaders from above while leading those below.

As your practice's administrator, what you can accomplish is directly dependent on how well your middle managers can perform, and how quickly they can grow and adapt to an ever-changing environment.

Every administrator has an individual approach to curating the management team, but it mostly amounts to informal, problem-focused efforts rather than proactive work. We suggest you become more formal and proactive, and this chapter may help.

Wohl C, Pinto JB. *UP: Taking Ophthalmic Administrators and Their Management Teams to the Next Level of Skill, Performance, and Career Satisfaction, Second Edition* (pp 85-94). © 2021 Taylor & Francis Group.

This chapter contains a long, but by no means exhaustive, recap of the numerous possible dimensions of career development and performance improvement. These are broken down and arranged as a two-column tool. Feel free to edit and expand this tool liberally to fit your unique setting and the expectations you have for your team. You can use this tool to help take an already-strong manager to the next level, or to rescue a faltering manager.

Make photocopies of this tool for an extended sit-down meeting with each of your managers in turn. This paperwork will help you assess, support, nurture (and celebrate!) each manager's growth.

How to use this tool:

- Use the topical notes in the left-hand column to start a dialog with each middle manager. You can read the left-hand column together, and then go beyond what's written to discuss specifics that apply to your own setting.
- Then ask your manager, "How do you think you are doing in this area? What would you like to work on or improve in this dimension of your career here? How can I help?"
- Finally, use the right-hand column to record any resolutions on which you both agree. Check for progress periodically.

1. **Learning and understanding new business management concepts**

Topic	What I Resolve to Do in This Area
The best managers set aside time to read books, periodicals, and online resources that can enhance their understanding of management and business concepts. Such managers ask after each reading: "How could I apply these concepts in my role as a department manager?"	
The role of all managers is to extract the most value from the limited resources they are given. This principally involves staff resources but also extends to facilities, equipment, software, available training time, external experts, etc. What ideas do you have to extract more value from your available resources?	

2. **Human resources (HR) management**

Topic	What I Resolve to Do in This Area
Few practices are large enough to have a dedicated HR department. HR tasks are often split between the administrator and supervisors, with some clerical or outsourced help on the side. How are you doing in the role you have here to hire the right employees? To reassign or remove the wrong employees? How are you coming along on finding and fixing conflicts between staff? Do you think you set a good example for staff to follow? Do you adhere closely enough to policies?	

3. **Relationship building**

Topic	What I Resolve to Do in This Area
As a middle manager, you are at the center of numerous relationships with senior and junior staff, doctors, employees, vendors, and others. How well do you do at balancing all of these relationships? Do you put in enough time to maintain these relationships? Are any relationships frayed that you would like to improve?	

4. **Evolving management skills into leadership skills**

Topic	What I Resolve to Do in This Area
Managers administrate, leaders innovate. As a middle manager it is ideal to combine these roles. You have to follow existing rules. But you also have to be on the lookout for policies and procedures in need of a change. Are you equally a manager and a leader today? How might you develop more leadership skills? What steps could you take and how might I help you?	

5. **Problem solving**

Topic	What I Resolve to Do in This Area
Effective practice leaders look beyond surface symptoms. They find and cure the "problem behind the problem." Example: Patient volumes are down. Is it because of • Recall gaps? • Competition? • Failed customer service? • Contract loss? It is very tempting to jump to a solution before you truly understand the problem and the options. Avoid fixing just the symptom of the problem. Problems are often multidimensional and require collaboration to solve. How are you doing in your development as a problem solver?	

6. **Numeracy**

Topic	What I Resolve to Do in This Area
Like a doctor gathering lab data to treat patients, a manager needs to measure and track trends within a department. Numeracy is the number one skill that many managers wish they performed better. The skills needed to be good at the numbers in an ophthalmology practice require little more than basic math and a bit of memorization. Example: A general ophthalmology clinic sees 1200 visits per month. How many techs do they need to employ? Answer: The typical practice needs 1 hour of tech time per patient visit and there are 173 work hours in an average month. So the math is: (1200 pts x 1 hr) / 173 = 6.9 techs	

(continued)

Topic	What I Resolve to Do in This Area
This simple calculation is a sample of a key performance indicator (KPI). What KPIs are important to track in your department? Do you track them? What are the current values and how do these compare to norms? How would you like to develop your skills in this area? It is important to be familiar with reports that impact your department. These can include: • Staff productivity reports addition/subtraction/realignment • Revenue cycle management reports (eg, open accounts over 90 days) • Call center reports (eg, average talk time, abandoned call rate, average hold time) • Department budget Which reports are you expected to review? Do you understand them all or need additional tutorials? Are there additional reports or data you would like to receive? What is your plan for reviewing each of these daily? Weekly? Monthly?	

7. **Communication skills**

Topic	What I Resolve to Do in This Area
Communication skills are a key success factor to being an excellent manager. The following is a list of specific skills. Score yourself (1 to 10) for each one and develop specific "I will do this" goals for each low score. • Emails to staff and doctors • Policies and procedures • Regular use of written communication, in addition to verbal communication, rather than mostly verbal • Performance evaluations • Disciplinary documentation • Proposals and requests • Verbal clarity when speaking • Meeting presentations	

8. **Effective delegation**

Topic	What I Resolve to Do in This Area
Having others handle appropriate tasks, rather than doing it yourself, provides the opportunity to concentrate on higher-level responsibilities. Delegating provides others an opportunity to learn and grow, and should not be seen as dumping your work on others. List three things you could do better in delegating to others.	

9. **Organizational skills**

Topic	What I Resolve to Do in This Area
Being organized is critical for completing tasks in an efficient and effective manner, and to allow you to be a role model for the people you supervise. How are you doing at keeping yourself organized? How well do you manage your: • Desk and work areas • To-do lists (daily, weekly, monthly) • Calendar • Other What do you need to do to improve? List one or two things you might commit to trying for 1 month.	

10. **Prioritization skills**

Topic	What I Resolve to Do in This Area
Do you spend major time on major things or get distracted by less important items? Are your priorities in line with those of the overall practice? Do you hold yourself accountable for deadlines? What would you like to improve in this area?	

11. **Time management**

Topic	What I Resolve to Do in This Area
Every manager reports, "There is not enough time in the day!" Time management is affected by many of the skills already reviewed here (delegation, prioritization, and organization skills). What else can you do to improve your time management?	

12. **Customer service**

Topic	What I Resolve to Do in This Area
Patient expectations continue to rise. Department managers are on the front lines of customer care. They set and uphold company-wide performance standards. What are you doing in your department to evaluate and address customer service gaps? Is this topic a regular agenda item for department meetings? How quickly are patient complaints addressed? Whose responsibility is it to do so? If not yours, is the line of communication adequate so whoever needs to respond to patients is notified quickly? What ideas do you have to improve the customer service that your department provides?	

13. **Making the difficult transition from being an equal peer in your department to being the department's supervisor**

Topic	What I Resolve to Do in This Area
Moving from being a co-worker to being a department manager is a big challenge. Not only are you learning new skills and have a brand new job description, but you are contending with former peers who may be jealous, angry, or unsupportive. Peer-to-peer friendships often suffer. Working with your administrator can help to diminish problems in this area. What can I do to help you through any lingering transition issues?	

14. **Running effective meetings**

Topic	What I Resolve to Do in This Area
Meetings are a fact of life when you are a leader. What challenges do you face when running a meeting? Are the frequency, duration, and content correct? Do you prepare and distribute an agenda and meeting minutes? Does your agenda include problem-solving opportunities in addition to sharing information? Is there anything I could do as administrator to assist you in this area (eg, coaching, attending or not attending certain meetings, backing up your directives better)?	

15. **Following through and being action-oriented**

Topic	What I Resolve to Do in This Area
Managers not only have to perform tasks and assign tasks to others, they also have to ensure that all of the tasks are completed. How are you performing in this key area? Are all tasks completed on time, or do some slip through the cracks? What could you do to be better at follow-through and keeping yourself and staff accountable?	

16. **Written operational guidelines for the department**

Topic	What I Resolve to Do in This Area
Operations manuals memorialize the "one, agreed-upon, best" way to do everything. An operations manual forces service consistency and reduces errors and costly mistakes. It also formalizes staff training, which advances quality improvement. Do you have an up-to-date operations manual for each area of your department's responsibility? Do you add a policy or procedure each time a new problem arises that you solve for the first time? How might you take this dimension of your career to the next level of performance?	

17. **Seeking assistance when difficult challenges arise**

Topic	What I Resolve to Do in This Area
No manager is an island. If you are a newer manager, you may not yet fully understand what you don't know. Regularly held meetings with your administrator provide the opportunity to explore novel solutions and help you recognize knowledge deficits. Do you readily ask for help, or could you do a better job at asking for assistance?	

18. **Understanding and complying with regulatory demands**

Topic	What I Resolve to Do in This Area
As a provider of critical medical care, as an employer, and especially as a federal contractor, our practice is subject to thousands of regulations, many more than the typical business. Accordingly, we all have to know and respect the rules, and look in our individual departments and beyond for any areas where our compliance may be lapsing. Do you know the key regulations that apply to your department? Are you aware of any regulations where our practice is not fully compliant? (And if you noticed something problematic, would you feel comfortable coming forward to report the problem to management or the board?)	

CHAPTER 17

Begin With the Ending in Mind

What Level of Management Staff Does Your Practice Need to Succeed in the Future?

The way a team plays as a whole determines its success. You may have the greatest bunch of individual stars in the world, but if they don't play together, the club won't be worth a dime.
—Babe Ruth

Senior management is simply a flag bearer when a business decision is made. It is of no use unless others follow the flag.
—Eiji Toyota

As regulatory complexities rise, profits soften and the size of the average practice increases, there is an increasing obligation to deepen the skills of your practice's management team. Most practices do this basic business development work haphazardly, not by plan.

Why is this a common trend we see? Because the practice and its leaders are so focused on building the patient base, providing excellent care, honing finances, and hiring staff and doctors to keep up with the volume that just having enough managers can be the focus, rather than ensuring that your managers have all the skills you need in your current environment.

Wohl C, Pinto JB. *UP: Taking Ophthalmic Administrators and Their Management Teams to the Next Level of Skill, Performance, and Career Satisfaction, Second Edition* (pp 95-98). © 2021 Taylor & Francis Group.

The following are hallmarks in ophthalmic practices that report feeling in control of whatever may arise in the future for their organizations.

A Lack of Dependency on Any One Manager

"Our administrator could be away from the practice for a month or two, and the practice would keep on running just fine. The administrator has empowered our department heads to make their own decisions, and has worked with the managing partner so the lead doctor can step in and handle any senior management issues while the administrator is away. In addition, each department has a 'second lieutenant' so that even if the department head is out of the office, someone is clearly in charge and keeping operations on track."

Some managers feel threatened by this lack of short-term dependency, but in reality, it can strengthen your position in the company because you are freer to spend time working on higher-valued responsibilities. The only way to climb your career ladder is by leaving behind the rungs below you.

Written Process Documentation

"Everything we do here is put down in writing. There is one, agreed-upon, best way to check in a patient, take a history, and work our open insurance accounts. This makes training easier, and when staffers grasp their job duties faster, they are easier to supervise. At the same time, everyone in our practice is encouraged to propose a better way for any of our protocols."

No Managers on Overload

"If you observed our department heads and administrator in action, they have a calm, in-control demeanor. They prioritize and pace their work, and delegate avidly so they always have reserve capacity for the inevitable emergencies."

Being the calm in the storm goes a long way in practice management. It adds stability and strength to the management team. And calm, collected managers are viewed as leaders, which is what your want in your practice.

Strategic Intimacy

"Our board is very aligned about the future direction our practice is taking. And they have shared their strategic plan with the entire management team, so everyone knows the operational priorities and volumetric goals. In addition, the board listens to us, and makes sure that plans for the practice are not getting out ahead of what the company can reasonably accomplish."

As consultant and quality guru Joseph M. Juran said, "Without a standard, there is no logical basis for decision making or taking action." Providing the management team and all staff with your goals and standards provides the guidance they need to make good decisions.

Job Tenure

"The average manager has been in our practice for more than a decade. They know what great operations look like, and how to turn things around when they get off track. Because of our managers' knowledge and tenure, the staff they supervise—as well as the doctors—trust their skills. With the doctors in particular, this sets up a virtuous cycle: more tenure leads to greater skills ... and greater skills lead to higher trust by the board ... and more trust leads to greater job satisfaction and longer careers."

• • •

How does your practice compare with these optimal hallmarks? How do YOU stack up? Here is an exercise to help you identify—specifically and practically, rather than just theoretically—where the holes might be in your management team.

Creating the Management Team You Need

1. Gather the administrator and practice owners. Set a timer for 30 minutes. With this artificial deadline, brainstorm as a group where the practice will be in 5 years. Include answers to these questions:
   a. What will be our service area (the north/west/south/east boundaries for our operations)?
   b. How many office locations will we have?
   c. In the next 5 years, what patient services will we add/subtract?
   d. What will be our annual collections? Patient visit counts? Surgery counts?
   e. How fast will we be growing? (Note: The average practice today is growing about 4% per year.)
   f. How many doctors, of what type, will we have?
   g. How many staff will we employ in each department?

Don't try to create a polished strategic planning document with this exercise. Just write down random thoughts arising around the table. Even if some of these thoughts are in conflict or if there is an emerging difference of opinion, these can be ironed out in subsequent drafts.

2. Continue your brainstorming by writing down as many details as you can about how your management team will need to adapt to this future plan over time. Here are some questions to consider:
   a. Will we have the same administrator, or will a new senior staffer be required (either because of retirement or a gap in needed skills that may arise with practice growth)?
   b. What will be the job scope and role of the managing partner of the practice?
   c. What gaps in basic management team structure and organization do we need to fill? Does every manager have a formal position description? Are reporting lines clear or blurred? Are there annual (or more frequent) performance assessments? Are meetings held with appropriate frequency and follow-up?
   d. Whether the practice is static or growing, what new skills will be needed generally in the middle management cohort? A clearer understanding of human resources law? Deeper financial skills? Formal supervisory training? Time available? Career commitment? What new skills will be needed department-by-department?
3. Finally, write down what action should be taken in the next 12 months to prepare the management team for where the practice is heading 5 years from now. Here are some examples from other practice settings:
   a. Recruit a new director of technical services to replace our retiring director.
   b. Establish a project tracker so that each new project or initiative has a clear owner and deadline.
   c. Designate an assistant manager for the patient accounts department so that when the manager is away from the practice the staff has a clear supervisor in place.
   d. Hold management team meetings biweekly instead of monthly, and make sure the managing partner is present for at least half of these.
   e. Find a more private office for our administrator so they are not constantly being interrupted, and so sensitive paperwork can be kept out and worked on throughout the day.

CHAPTER 18

Peer-to-Supervisor Promotions

Transitions and Challenges

Often the best solution to a management problem is the right person.
—Edwin Booz

As a business owner or manager, you know that hiring the wrong person is the most costly mistake you can make.
—Brian Tracy

All progress takes place outside the comfort zone.
—Michael John Bobak

The majority of ophthalmic practices in the country are small, with a handful of providers. For practices at this scale, a typical organizational chart includes one doctor-leader, one administrator, and two or three supervisors.

How many mid-level managers or working supervisors (and what kind) are needed for your practice depends on several variables:

- How departmentalized is the practice?
- Are there ambulatory surgical centers or optical ancillaries?
- How many locations are present?
- How fast is the practice growing?
- How hands-on or delegating is the administrator?
- Are the physician-owners involved with business management?

Wohl C, Pinto JB. *UP: Taking Ophthalmic Administrators and Their Management Teams to the Next Level of Skill, Performance, and Career Satisfaction, Second Edition* (pp 99-103).

Your practice's leaders—administrators, middle managers, and supervisors—often begin their careers as entry-level billers, techs, or receptionists. With hard work and an aptitude for managing others, they climb their way up the ladder.

But sometimes the rungs can break.

Some new managers, after hard work and effort to advance, are held back from their full leadership potential because they find it difficult to shift from being a peer to being the boss.

In this chapter, we will focus on the typical challenges that occur when you promote an employee to be a working supervisor or manager. But first, let's discuss how you can better identify potential new supervisors within your practice from among the rank and file.

In most practices, great potential leaders are hiding in plain sight. It's not unusual for a client to say, "We really don't have any techs who would make an acceptable department supervisor." But when we interview the techs individually, one or two great candidates inevitably surface. What do we seek?

At the top of the list, you look for the competency in the core skills of the candidate's current position and that the candidate is respected among peers for being among the most skilled in the department. This doesn't necessarily align with tenure. Some excellent supervisors are selected who are by no means the most senior in their department. Several other traits should be visible:

- Prioritization, organization, and time management
- A collaborating spirit (not a glory hog)
- Being proactive
- Good at building work relationships
- A natural, persistent, problem solver
- Expresses appreciation to others
- Accepts blame, when appropriate
- Strong, comfortable communication skills
- Someone you will feel comfortable taking into your confidence and discussing sensitive matters
- Already acts as an informal leader among peers in their department
- Makes potentially unpopular suggestions for the good of the patients or practice
- Contributes toward productivity, likes to keep working when others rest
- Accomplishes less with more
- Speaks up and advocates for the department appropriately

In the best of situations, you may have two equally qualified members of a department as candidates. How do you choose? One approach is to let the two finalists decide between themselves who the next department head should be. The person who wants it the most will almost always be selected, and with leadership, it's often the person who most wants to lead who ends up being the most effective. (You never want to draft an unwilling department member to head the department, no matter how skilled at their core job.)

If you're still stuck between two internal candidates, you can test the waters by giving each finalist an assignment or task as a fitness test:

- Lead a departmental brainstorming session
- Participate on an interdepartmental task force
- Present an educational segment at a staff meeting

Be open-minded and creative in your approach when it comes to considering internal candidates. Candidates with a strong desire and ambition to succeed, as long as they have some of the skill sets needed, may surprise you.

The fear of failure and being demoted back to a nonsupervisory employee status can cloud the judgment of a potential candidate who may decline the opportunity. You can offer the new position in the acting capacity, which makes a retreat easier. All the same, make sure your final candidate is not accepting the position offered simply to make the administrator or doctors happy.

Let's turn now to the most common struggle that can emerge when you make a rank-and-file member of a department the department lead: adjusting from being a peer to being a boss.

It generally takes at least 12 months to shake the jealousy and some testing of the new manager. This common testing of the new manager's authority is typically not undertaken by all members of the department, but only by a few people, either co-workers who had become personal friends, or co-workers who were already nominally competitive with the new manager back when they were peers.

Occasionally, the new manager will have to terminate a staffer who just can't accept the change and is too much of a pot-stirrer to keep employed.

Workplace relationships, even in the absence of the natural friendships that arise, are tricky. But working relationships are harmed when rank-and-file department members remain personally friendly when one of them is promoted. One of the hardest things for a new up-through-the-ranks manager to do is to revise old friendships and create a bit of professional distance between worker and boss. Here are some things you can say as an administrator to the mid-level manager you have just promoted to help get through this common adjustment:

1. Favoritism has the same result on a team, whether its perception or reality. Even if you think you are being fair and unbiased, your decisions and actions will always be questioned.
2. You might ultimately have to hold your friend to a higher standard, being stricter with expectations, to counter the perception of favoritism. (Like being the coach of your daughter's softball team, where kids with less talent may be played more, so it doesn't appear that your own child is favored.)
3. Emotions can impact your decision making, consciously or unconsciously. It may appear in scheduling, assignments, promotions, and raises.
4. Your employee-friend could have unrealistic or unprofessional expectations of you, expecting you to share confidential information or get favored treatment. This could make you feel uncomfortable and, ultimately, such friendships unwind in disappointing and hurtful ways, so its better to unwind them when you become a supervisor.

5. Your feelings will be hurt. Most employees will find something to complain about with their peers, even about the best managers. Peer pressure will win, especially if your friend does not want to be perceived to be favored. You will surely hear about it, and you could take it more personally than if another employee had the same complaint.
6. Managers are supposed to be role models. If you maintain this role while outside the office with an employee, it may feel inauthentic and would be less fun for you. If you lose the manager persona for a few hours after work, it's harder for you to regain it while at work.
7. Other employees may expect you to not take action on issues that involve your friend, so they won't provide you with potentially important information about shortcomings or errors happening at work. You won't find out about them until the gaps are wide and upper management will (appropriately) hold you responsible.

As hard as it is to do, every human resources professional's wisdom is applicable in situations like this: avoid being friends with your work subordinates.

So what does the new manager do about old friends?

The common advice is that you can be friendly, warm, caring, supportive, have fun together, but not friends. You can go to an after-work happy hour to be social, but make it a habit to leave after the first drink and not be around when everyone else lets their hair down. Avoid being in the Facebook photos, especially as a protection to yourself and the practice. Should something go awry, there won't be the perception that it was a company-approved function or management's responsibility.

As difficult as it may be, unfriend your employees on Facebook and stop getting together outside of work. Boundaries between supervisors and employees need to be established and followed. If you want to be a successful and professional manager, stepping back from friendships is the painful best policy. True friends, those who want the best for you, will understand that the transition is necessary.

• • •

Here are some fast tips for selecting an internal candidate for promotion and the skills they need to have or development to make the leap from worker to working supervisor.

Supervising for Success: Tips for Brand New Supervisors

Skill sets needed:

1. Organization and planning
   a. Organize your thoughts.
   b. Plan for the outcome you want.
2. Communication
   a. Set expectations, in writing and while speaking at meetings.
   b. Listening, the art of listening, is important for successful problem solving
   c. Feedback goes both ways. Be prepared to hear what your former peers think of you and your ideas. It's not personal but may feel that way.

3. Be approachable
   a. Open to criticism
   b. Not defensive
   c. Humble
   d. Viewed as part of the team
4. Time management: Approach tasks and responsibilities with efficiency and streamline your goals
5. Prioritize: Spend your limited management time on what aligns with overall practice goals
6. Confrontation (the good kind)
   a. Address issues promptly.
   b. Be fearless. It works out best in the end.
   c. Focus on the big picture of the department or practice, not individuals only.
7. Objectivity: Avoid the perception of favoritism.

CHAPTER 19

Wohl's Rules for Building a Strong Mid-Level Management Team

If you can't fly, then run. If you can't run, then walk.
If you can't walk, then crawl, but whatever you do,
you have to keep moving forward.
— Martin Luther King, Jr.

If you spend any time in the gym, you know that core strength provides a base allowing you to move the rest of your body more powerfully. This applies not only at the gym, where arms and legs do their best when supported by a strong core, but also with the careers of your middle managers, who help to anchor your practice.

Great doctors and great administrators need great mid-level managers who can absorb and understand practice goals, and then frame up protocols to manage staff effectively and carry out the smallest operational details. Your middle managers are the critical core of your practice.

Wohl C, Pinto JB. *UP: Taking Ophthalmic Administrators and Their Management Teams to the Next Level of Skill, Performance, and Career Satisfaction, Second Edition* (pp 105-106).

But mid-level managers, especially in smaller practices, often get shortchanged when it comes to opportunities to learn and grow stronger as leaders. They need more of your time. More training resources. And often, much more positive feedback from providers.

As "working supervisors," mid-levels have so much to get done, there's not much time or energy left over for them to *get better* unless you help.

Here are 10 rules that will help to strengthen and align your middle managers.

Wohl's Rules for a Strong Mid-Level Management Team

1. Middle managers are the fundamental building blocks of your practice. No practice can be strong without a robust cohort of middle managers, even if you have the best doctors and the best administrator.
2. Some discomfort may be required to continuously improve your team. Constant progress is crucial. Small steps. Keep up the momentum, push goals, expectations.
3. Know each manager's limits and keep taking them right up to the edge of their limits.
4. Help managers be eager learners. Carve out time for study and thinking, not only doing. Provide access to educational materials and time to learn.
5. Select a manager who desires the position and will be energized by the challenge. Especially, pick people who exhibit energy, curiosity, and excitement to dig in and solve problems.
6. Each important department head needs a second lieutenant, a #2 in charge. Your practice needs depth on the bench to avoid being vulnerable to changes you cannot control. Make you and your practice invulnerable to loss of management staff.
7. Push decision making aggressively down the chain of command. To do otherwise means your managers do not develop the confidence, skills, or independence to run their departments. The administrator will constantly need to drop back to handle small issues, which distracts from senior executive duties.
8. Give your management team abundant credit. In turn, they will pass credit down to their line staff.
9. Weigh facts and feelings equally as you manage your middle managers. You can't just feel your way to the best decisions. You also have to calculate your way.
10. Put everything in writing. Everything. Management's chief job is to decide, document, and communicate with clarity throughout the practice.

Section IV

Ophthalmology Is a Team Sport

CHAPTER 20

How Aligned Is Our Practice?

You have to decide what your highest priorities are and have the courage—pleasantly, smilingly, nonapologetically—to say "no" to other things. And the way to do that is by having a bigger "YES" burning inside.
—Stephen Covey

Any intelligent fool can make things bigger and more complex. It takes a touch of genius—and a lot of courage—to move in the opposite direction.
—Albert Einstein

In life, as in football, you won't go far unless you know where the goalposts are.
—Arnold H. Glasgow

Successful coaches, business owners, and managers agree: only when a team is aligned and in sync can it effectively achieve an organization's objectives ... whether the team is a business or a sports franchise. It takes a common vision of the desired outcome. It takes planning, communication, constant oversight, and monitoring. Everyone up and down the ranks must be held accountable to the goals. When we get the big picture straight, the details are more likely to be on target.

Wohl C, Pinto JB. *UP: Taking Ophthalmic Administrators and Their Management Teams to the Next Level of Skill, Performance, and Career Satisfaction, Second Edition* (pp 109-113). © 2021 Taylor & Francis Group.

Let's apply this concept to a winning professional football team. Everyone on the team knows, from the owner to the kids handing out Gatorade, what they want and what they need:

- We want to be the #1 team at the end of the season.
- To be #1, we have to win more games than the other teams.
- To win more games, we have to play better than the other teams.
- To play better, we have to have the best athletes available and make the best plays.
- To have the best athletes and plays, we need money, scouts, coaches, trainers, and an owner willing to provide these needed resources.

Is your practice similarly aligned? Does your team want to win? Are your owners aware of what that takes and willing to supply the needed resources?

Below are questions for the management team and board of directors alike to help you evaluate how aligned your practice is and what you need to do for better alignment.

How Aligned Is Our Practice?

Areas of potential alignment or misalignment for the administrator, department heads, and partners to discuss	Our current alignment score *0=Poor* *10=Excellent*	Actions we could take to improve this score (eg, "agree to disagree," "write down a firm policy," "seek a third opinion")
Are the owners and managers on the same page about the long-term planning for the practice: How fast to grow? Service area? Provider mix? Services to add or subtract?		
Does the pace and tempo and work intensity of the management team align with the ambitions and pacing of the board? (Ideally, the managers are not lagging behind the board's desired intensity, nor should the management team get too far ahead of the board.)		
What is our philosophy about individual scope of practice: Should every doctor practice as they please or be obliged to perform services that best serve the practice's institutional interests?		

(continued)

How Aligned Is Our Practice? (continued)

Areas of potential alignment or misalignment for the administrator, department heads, and partners to discuss	**Our current alignment score** *0=Poor* *10=Excellent*	**Actions we could take to improve this score (eg, "agree to disagree," "write down a firm policy," "seek a third opinion")**
What is our philosophy about support staff protocols, particularly technicians? Are the protocols individually defined by the physician or is there one best agreed-upon policy for each work task that makes it easier for staff to be assigned and work efficiently for any and all physicians and office locations?		
Do we have quality of care standards and what are they: Are providers in our practice expected to provide average care or better? Top 10% care?		
Profit vs quality: Should profit come foremost or should profit take a back seat to the quality and sophistication of services rendered (eg, the latest equipment, abundance of staff)?		
External relationships: Who are our friends and competitors?		
Risk management: What risks (eg, financial, clinical, reputational) are reasonable to take?		
Utilization: Are our surgeons on the same page with respect to surgical assertiveness, testing rates, etc? Do we want to set standards or monitoring guidelines?		

(continued)

How Aligned Is Our Practice? (continued)

Areas of potential alignment or misalignment for the administrator, department heads, and partners to discuss	Our current alignment score *0=Poor* *10=Excellent*	Actions we could take to improve this score (eg, "agree to disagree," "write down a firm policy," "seek a third opinion")
Ethical compass: Do the partners have similar/compatible ethical standards?		
Profit apportionment: How much profit should be distributed to physicians vs being reinvested in the business? Do we have agreed-upon policy that helps us make fair reinvestment decisions?		
Physician compensation modeling: Does the comp model fairly apportion profits between the partners (including locums profits)? Do we revisit and either confirm or revise the comp model every 2 years?		
Mutuality: To what degree do partners have each other's backs and trust each other? To what degree does the management team have each other's backs and trust each other? Are managers expected to offer help "beyond department lines" for the benefit of all patients and practice reputation?		
Outside activities: To what degree are partners allowed to pursue outside clinical or business interests?		

(continued)

How Aligned Is Our Practice? (continued)

Areas of potential alignment or misalignment for the administrator, department heads, and partners to discuss	**Our current alignment score** *0=Poor* *10=Excellent*	**Actions we could take to improve this score (eg, "agree to disagree," "write down a firm policy," "seek a third opinion")**
Power and decision sharing: Is control balanced fairly among the partners?		
Facilities, staff, promotion, and equipment: Do partners have reasonable access to these needed resources? Are departments and managers supported equally for needed space and equipment?		
Other:		
Other:		

CHAPTER 21

Leading Your Team Past the Inevitable Conflicts of Practice Life

Whenever you're in conflict with someone, there is one factor that can make the difference between damaging your relationship and deepening it. That factor is attitude.
—William James

Courage is what it takes to stand up and speak. Courage is also what it takes to sit down and listen.
—Winston Churchill

You can choose courage, or you can choose comfort, but you cannot choose both.
—Brené Brown

When leading others, even in the most genteel of practices, two simple truths apply that you need to master. First, conflicts will always occur, even among the kindest, best-intentioned individuals in a work group. And second, the excellence of your leadership is not measured by how few conflicts arise on your watch, but by how quickly and effectively these conflicts are reduced and resolved by you.

Practice conflicts have always been prominent when leading in this people-intensive arena. These conflicts arise from the host of innate personalities found in those who gravitate to medicine. The adverse behaviors flowing from these personalities are now magnified in an environment of progressively tighter finances and sharply clearer threats to business survival.

Wohl C, Pinto JB. *UP: Taking Ophthalmic Administrators and Their Management Teams to the Next Level of Skill, Performance, and Career Satisfaction, Second Edition* (pp 115-119).

However, in most clinic settings, conflict is not diffuse and generalized. We can often point to one "PITA" who is an enduring wellspring of conflict. We are not referring to the Mediterranean flat bread, here, but the acronym for a "pain in the rump." It's likely that one person in your practice is your major annoyance and a distraction to your leadership responsibilities. This can be a provider, a lay staff member, or increasingly, if you work in a corporate health system or multispecialty clinic, an institutional colleague or overseer.

We are all periodically a PITA, even the angels among us. Durable PITAs are the greater challenge. The adverse impact of workplace PITAs is magnified by leaders who fail to lay down and enforce strong rules, or in settings where roles are unclear and there are unintended signals sent to your office PITA that it's okay to buck authority and make others miserable.

In the same way that parents are responsible for calming family conflicts issuing from their children, it is the responsibility of the more senior practice leaders—owners and managers—to resolve conflicts occurring at lower levels. Just as an effective physician reveals a disease and applies the appropriate treatment briskly, the effective practice leader finds and fixes conflict without delay. Everyone involved in a conflict needs to be called into the room at the earliest possible moment. However, unlike disease managers, business managers can be conflict avoidant and uncertain how to start the discussion. You may, though, be personally comfortable taking action if the decision is completely yours, but reticent to do so because you are unsure your doctor-leaders will support your action.

In heated settings it can help to draw a conflict diagram to stimulate a group dialog and better understand who "owns" a conflict. Envision a conflict scale of 0 to 10. A 0 means the complete absence of conflict. When two people have a conflict level of 10 it's hard for them to be in the same room, much less work productively with each other.

Almost no workplace pairings are at a 0. A low-grade, benign struggle in the range of 1 to 3 occurs naturally, even between people who work well together. This low-grade struggle can spike at times and reach conflict levels of, let's say, 5 or 6, which is somewhat uncomfortable. If the conflict level stays this high for weeks, months, or longer it can negatively impact the practice and the individuals exposed to the conflict.

Fortunately, most people are reasonable, and, disliking how it feels to be in conflict with another person, willing to talk it over, work it out without any outside help, and drop back to a 2 or 3 again. When two people have a hard time walking a conflict back, it may indicate the need to bring in a third person. Even the happiest couples, in the course of a long marriage, can benefit from a session here and there with a counselor, clergy, or trusted relative. In a business setting, difficult conflicts between doctors or staff members are walked back by a similar third party—an administrator, doctor, a consultant, or industrial psychologist, or, in the toughest settings, the practice's attorney.

Sometimes conflicts are simple and dyadic—involving only two people in the practice. At other times, conflicts can be complex to understand, much less resolve. A tool we use in our work is a conflict diagram.

In the simple diagram shown, Dave, Mike, and Mary are three eye surgeons, partners in their group practice. Mike and Mary have a very low level of conflict with each other—a 2 as marked on the diagram. Dave and Mike have a high level of conflict, at an 8. Dave and Mary have an even stronger level of conflict, a 9.

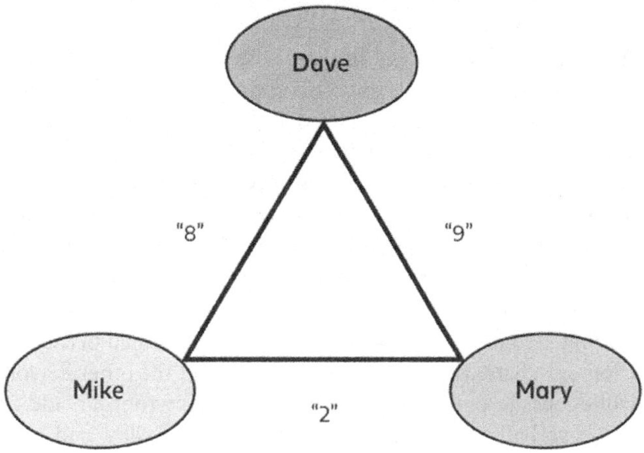

It's a good hunch in this setting that Dave could be the source of the conflict. A diagram like this is especially useful when you have more than three parties and are trying to communicate with your practice's PITA why you believe they could be chiefly responsible for the difficulty.

You can diagram and examine conflicts in your own practice in the same way. Write down the involved parties—this may be a cohort of doctors or the members of a single department. Array the names at the corners of a triangle (for three people), the corners of a square (for four people), and so forth. Then draw lines between each of the pairs and label each line based on your subjectively judged paired scores for their present level of conflict between each person on a 0 (low) to 10 (high) level. When finished, this diagram can be a useful basis for group or individual discussion. If you are a department head, you should feel comfortable addressing staff-to-staff conflicts in your department, or at least feel comfortable asking your administrator to step in as a moderator. As an administrator you probably feel comfortable refereeing a conflict between two mid-level managers. If you feel uncomfortable mediating a doctor-to-doctor conflict in your practice—which is a very reasonable feeling to have, especially if both parties are partners—you should call on the help of your managing partner, the board at large, or an outside facilitator.

• • •

Here are a few insights on conflict resolution abstracted from the writings of Richard Darlington, an eclectic British-Italian trade union negotiator, framed in an ophthalmic context.

1. **Be calm**. Conflict usually engenders strong emotions, even anger, but in such a state you are unlikely to be rational or in the mood for compromise. If two conflicting doctors are highly charged emotionally, take a time out and return to resolution efforts at another time.
2. **Show respect**. However much you disagree with a staff member or provider, try to attack the argument, not the person. This approach can break down when dealing with individuals who are themselves disrespectful of the discussion process. In such situations, group pressure or removal of the offending party from a group discussion are the common resorts used by effective leaders.
3. **Be magnanimous**. In truth, most conflict is over matters of little substance, and often it is mostly pride or status that is at stake. Consider conceding the point to your opponent, just as an effective martial arts practitioner steps aside rather than absorb a blow. And don't hold a grudge.
4. **Discuss or debate**. So often, conflict is created or maintained because there is no real discussion or debate. We make assumptions about the other person's point of view and willingness to compromise, which might be wrong. In addition to discussing an issue verbally, diagram it on a whiteboard or yellow pad.
5. **Be rational**. Much conflict is not about substance but perception. Try to work through mere perception to discover and agree on how things really are. Ophthalmology is a fact-laden enterprise, the management of an ophthalmic practice should be similarly factual and rational. Use benchmarks, industry standards and the documentation of the best-demonstrated practices to agree on what's true, before trying to hammer out disagreements.
6. **Acknowledge emotions**. Facts alone, however rational, sometimes cannot resolve a conflict because how people perceive those facts is colored by their emotions. It's no good denying those emotions, so make an effort to see the situation the way the other person does and to acknowledge their emotions before endeavoring to move beyond them. Use phrases such as "Please allow me to explain why this is so important to me."
7. **Change the wording**. It's amazing how often we disagree about words and how a change of words can alter how people view a situation. Instead of criticizing a young associate for his low surgical volumes, invite him to set future growth goals, backed up by new outreach efforts.
8. **Change the environment**. It's no coincidence that some of the toughest political negotiations of all times, for instance those that were aimed at Middle East peace, often took place in serene, neutral locations like the Camp David presidential retreat. Don't hold tough board meetings in the staff lounge. Reserve a private dining room at everyone's favorite restaurant or borrow your attorney's boardroom.
9. **Consider sequencing**. Much conflict is created and aggravated by lack of trust. Building trust takes time and proof of goodwill. Consider introducing an agreement in stages with progression toward the ultimate goal.

10. **Seek mediation**. This is a process whereby a neutral third party consults with those involved in a conflict to see if the problem can be presented in a way that facilitates a resolution. The mediator may simply listen and ask questions or suggest other ways of looking at the problem or proposed solutions.
11. **If absolutely necessary, apply your authority**. Conflict can sometimes only be resolved by one party imposing his or her authority as the department head, administrator, or managing partner. Such a forced settlement may cause resentment for the nominal losers but sometimes this is the only way to resolve a conflict and move on.
12. **If all else fails, wait**. Most problems change over time. Either the problem solves itself because circumstances change or one's attitude about the problem changes as the heat dies down and other practice matters assume more prominence.

Adapted from Darlington R. How to resolve conflict. Modified April 18, 2007. Accessed March 12, 2021. http://www.rogerdarlington.co.uk/conflict.html

CHAPTER 22

How to Lead More Effective Meetings

You may be worried about earning their respect, and that's natural. Unfortunately, though, being overly focused on respect can backfire because it'll make you feel extra defensive when criticized. If, on the other hand, you can listen to the criticism and react well to it, both trust and respect will follow.
—Kim Malone Scott

Time—the one asset none of us are ever going to get more of.
—Gary Vaynerchuk

Even for the most competent ophthalmic administrators on the planet, leading a masterful, efficient, riveting, effective meeting is a skill you will never perfect, but one you will want to continue to improve throughout your career.

We all start out by learning the basics of running a meeting. With further thought and intention, mentoring—and abundant errors—we start to apply emotional intelligence and higher leadership skills to each meeting situation. We set the goal to make each meeting a productive, problem-solving, cohesion-building session. And we fall just a little short, until the next time.

In the following sections, you will find basic and advanced tips for running different types of meetings, but first, ask yourself these questions about each type of meeting you now schedule:

Wohl C, Pinto JB. *UP: Taking Ophthalmic Administrators and Their Management Teams to the Next Level of Skill, Performance, and Career Satisfaction, Second Edition* (pp 121-124). © 2021 Taylor & Francis Group.

- Is this meeting necessary, or is it mostly for announcements or something we could accomplish with a fact sheet, memo, or email?
- What is the cost of this meeting, and will the benefit exceed the cost? (A 1-hour meeting of five managers and the managing partner may represent $500 or more in labor.)
- Do we invite all the people needed at the meeting?
- Are we inviting people who don't really need to attend?
- Is the meeting duration, location, and start time optimal?
- Do we have the discipline of an agenda and notes memorializing what was decided?
- Do we generally emerge from these meetings with a sense of accomplishment?
- If this is a standing meeting (eg, a monthly board meeting), do we make linear progress or do we tend to keep revisiting old items over and over?
- Am I needed at this meeting or can I delegate my attendance to someone else?
- Even if this meeting is efficient and effective, what could we do to take it to the next level?

Better One-on-One Meetings (With Staff, Providers)

1. Quips to the contrary notwithstanding, all business is personal. Build rapport by being (appropriately) personally, genuinely interested ("How was your family vacation last week? How are you feeling after having the flu?").
2. Be prepared. Know the history. Don't rely on your memory. Look back in your notes to see where important discussions last left off. (Some managers keep a paper or electronic file on each person they work with closely, so they can remember from week to week what was last discussed or remember new topics to bring up at the next meeting.)
3. Let people know in advance what you expect from the meeting so they arrive prepared with:
   a. Updates on the slated discussion topics
   b. Follow up on the information from previously assigned tasks
   c. Their own agenda items or questions
4. Keep your own follow-up notes. Review these prior to any follow-up meetings.
5. Ask for feedback (eg, "Is there anything I could be doing more, less, or differently to be more effective on this matter?").
6. Ask questions like:
   a. Are there any barriers preventing you from achieving this?
   b. Are you waiting for me or others to provide you with anything you need to complete this assignment?

Tips for a More Motivating Managers' Meeting

1. Unless the wheels have completely fallen off, and everyone in the room is responsible, don't use management meetings to chastise or reprimand. These meetings should be 99% upbeat.
2. Stay optimistic. A positive company culture starts with you at the top of the management tier and rolls downward. Start by going around the room and expressing your gratitude to each attendee specifically about something you have been pleased seeing happen since the last meeting ("Mary, I've never seen the front desk neater or better organized, you are really whipping things into shape up there.").
3. Go around the room again allowing each manager a chance to share a departmental update and to report on open projects.
4. Be efficient with your time, but don't rush unduly. One of the great values of meeting with your management team is to foster a sense of belonging. It can be a pretty heavy load for some department heads to be the boss. They will do their best work with support from a group of managerial peers.
5. Teach something new at each meeting. Prepare a syllabus of general management concepts you would like the team to learn in the months ahead. As administrator, you can present some of these topics (a 10- to 15-minute brief in-service and discussion will generally suffice), and you can delegate some topics for presentation by the appropriate managers. Share articles that reinforce the topic. End each in-service by asking, "Does this teach us anything we could be doing around here?"
6. Adjourn, again, by being positive.

Preparing for and Conducting the Best Board Meetings

1. For most administrators, these are the highest-stakes meetings for your career, prepare accordingly.
2. The administrator and managing partner should co-prepare the agenda and should also prepare an attached one or two paragraph digest of the last month's and year-to-date financial and volumetric performance statistics for the practice.
3. In the typical setting, the managing partner opens the meeting with a few upbeat words of welcome and turns the gavel over to the administrator. At the end of the meeting, the administrator returns the gavel to the managing partner, who again says a few upbeat words in closing. In some settings, the managing partner runs the meeting.
4. At all times, the managing partner and administrator should be seen as a dyadic leadership pairing, on the same page, united, with no undue public disagreements.
5. Always, always, always use Robert's Rules of Order to run the meeting (with the formal, familiar motion-discussion-vote pattern … if you are unfamiliar with Robert's Rules, Google the Wikipedia entry and change your life).

6. As each topic comes up on the agenda, it will fall into just one of four simple categories:
   a. Announcement ("Dr. Smith has accepted her employment contract.")
   b. Decision today ("I move that we approve the purchase of a new OCT.")
   c. Decision in the future ("The building task force will review repaving bids and make a recommendation for the board to vote on at our next meeting.")
   d. Table ("Because our budget for the balance of the fiscal year is unclear, we will table until January a decision about setting up three new exam rooms.")
7. Move briskly and decide into which of these four categories a topic falls. Don't make the rookie mistake of endlessly discussing a subject with insufficient information for decision making or rehashing a decision that has already been made.
8. All board members must vote at all times in alignment with their fiduciary responsibility to the company, not in line with their personal interests.
9. All nonunanimous board decisions need to be supported by all board members (even if the vote didn't go your way).
10. Boards need to establish voting rules in their operating agreements, which establishes a quorum, describes the number of votes needed to carry various kinds of decisions, and discusses how tied votes are handled.
11. Because it can be awkward for the administrator to admonish board members who misbehave during the meeting (by talking out of turn) or after the meeting (by grousing to staff about a vote they lost), the managing partner needs to be the "sergeant at arms" keeping owners in line.

Miscellaneous Meeting Tips

1. An agenda is required for nearly all meetings.
2. Distribute the agenda to all meeting attendees at least 24 hours prior to the meeting.
3. Determine the amount of time needed for each agenda item. Allot the time for each topic and stick to it. Stay on task/topic and redirect others politely, as needed. If this is a challenge in your setting, bring a stopwatch or set your phone alarm to help the group keep on task.
4. Don't fall into the trap of randomly setting 1-hour meetings. The meeting will expand into the time allotted if not managed with intention.
5. During the meeting, when presenting each agenda item, state your goal and the kind of outcome you want from the discussion (and require each presenter to do the same).
6. Assign follow-up items. One person must own the task, even if it will be a team effort. Include a deadline.
7. Write (or delegate the writing of) meeting minutes and distribute within 72 hours.
8. Use an accountability document, such as an action grid (see Chapter 16 for a sample) for easy follow-up and review at the next meeting. This document becomes part of the meeting agenda packet each time, saving not only meeting time but also helping to keep assignments on track and not lost in the shuffle.

CHAPTER 23

What Makes a Team ... Work?

Evaluate How Your Teamwork Is Doing

Teamwork is work done by several associates, with each doing a part but all subordinating personal prominence to the efficiency of the whole.
—Cambridge Dictionary

Every practice agrees with the concept that taking a team approach is a core requirement for providing great patient care. Most administrators work very hard in a day-to-day task sense to foster teamwork. But very few practice teams call a time out in the game to agree on just what constitutes superior teamwork, and to nail down missing elements.

During selected brainstorming sessions with especially bright managers and the doctors they serve, we've had a few hundred front-line players in this game of eye care describe what they think makes for great teamwork. The assessment tool that follows is the result of these discussions.

Wohl C, Pinto JB. *UP: Taking Ophthalmic Administrators and Their Management Teams to the Next Level of Skill, Performance, and Career Satisfaction, Second Edition* (pp 125-129). © 2021 Taylor & Francis Group.

Teamwork Self-Assessment

Part One

Here's a self-assessment you can fill out individually or complete as a group exercise to measure selected aspects of your group's teamwork. This list of attributes of great teamwork is by no means complete, and no practice could be expected to have high scores in all of these areas.

Score each item on this 40-point list based on the following scale:

5 = I strongly agree with this statement.

4 = I agree with this statement.

3 = I am neutral; I neither agree nor disagree with this statement.

2 = I disagree with this statement.

1 = I strongly disagree with this statement.

_____ 1. Everyone on our practice team understands the historical context of our organization and where we've come from.

_____ 2. We have a written plan so everyone knows where we are heading in the future; group goals are clear.

_____ 3. We understand the rules of the game and how to keep score. We play to win, and celebrate our wins, both large and small.

_____ 4. We communicate well with each other, and we are especially good at listening.

_____ 5. We all understand the roles ("positions") that everyone plays on the team.

_____ 6. As "players" on the same team, we show respect and appreciation for each other, up and down the ranks.

_____ 7. Managers in our practice personally demonstrate good teamwork to the rest of the team.

_____ 8. The doctors personally demonstrate good teamwork to the rest of the team.

_____ 9. We have fun and enjoy playing "the game" together as a group.

_____ 10. We reward staff at every level for their ideas, performance, skills, motivation of others, flexibility, willingness to try and risk failure, sharing, small improvement, etc.

_____ 11. We set standards and expectations for teamwork that are appropriate, with especially high standards for senior lay staff and partner doctors.

_____ 12. We are constantly developing a better group understanding of what the customer wants and making service improvements in this context.

_____ 13. We hold a common mission to serve and delight all of the fans in the stands: patients and their family members, payers, referring doctors, employees and their dependent family members, etc.

_____ 14. We organize enough social interaction among the lay staff and doctors to develop great relationships with each other.

_____ 15. We educate everyone on the basics of every job, not only so we'll be able to cross-cover job functions, but so that we can have greater empathy for our colleagues' work environment.

_____ 16. We have developed specific performance expectations and standards and hold each other to these; we have created an environment where we each feel accountable to the team.

_____ 17. We understand the minimum standards of customer service and work together to exceed them.

_____ 18. We have boosted our investment in information technology to improve communication and productivity, and to reduce the frustration that comes with using outdated tools.

_____ 19. All members of the team are open to the input and reciprocal coaching of their colleagues. Our doctors are open to receiving and following through on the coaching efforts of their managers. Our managers are open to receiving and following the coaching efforts of the doctors.

_____ 20. We have a playbook (eg, the written personnel manual, operations manual, care pathways).

_____ 21. We get the team "psyched up" and elevate every teammate's reasonable expectations and enthusiasm about winning.

_____ 22. To watch us in action for 30 minutes, you would think we look more like a synchronized group than a collection of individuals running off in different directions.

_____ 23. We maintain a tempo that everyone can reasonably follow.

_____ 24. We seek a steady increase in both the individual and the combined talents of the team; we work hard to improve weak links and give them a fair chance to improve.

_____ 25. We deal with each other with empathy; we don't make fun of weak links in the team but, instead, help them.

_____ 26. When a weak link on the team can't be improved, we are not hesitant to remove him or her.

_____ 27. We don't withhold difficult information or triangulate (eg, when Mike complains to Ann about Mary).

_____ 28. We support decisive leadership and insist that our leaders lead.

_____ 29. We foster effective and appropriate "followership," the ability of team members to rally around the leader, and we respect the leader's position always, even if, from time to time, we harbor concerns about the individual leader involved.

_____ 30. We are time sensitive, and don't dawdle once a course of action has been ordered.

_____ 31. We sacrifice for, and compromise with, each other.

_____ 32. We remember there is no "I" in "TEAM" and that TEAM stands for "Together Everyone Achieves More."

_____ 33. We each take responsibility, others can count on us.
_____ 34. We balance authority with responsibility and give our managers the authority they need to carry out their duties.
_____ 35. We take in all viewpoints and don't discount even the most outlandish ideas.
_____ 36. We are energetic and have great stamina.
_____ 37. We make everyone on the team feel important.
_____ 38. We play carefully to avoid harming ourselves, others, or the company.
_____ 39. When any of us have our feelings hurt, we work through it and still stay in the game; we don't withdraw or quit playing.
_____ 40. Everyone plays; nobody sits on the bench for very long.

Total Score: ____________

Add up your score. With 40 different attributes, and with up to 5 points each, there's a maximum score of 200. There is no objective scale that compares you to others, but this summary score can be a valuable internal baseline of your teamwork and can help point out areas to improve. If you are working on improvements, it might be interesting to repeat this scoring instrument again in 6 months or 1 year.

Part Two

In addition to specific attributes of teamwork that you've measured above, it might be interesting to know what you think is the level of teamwork going on in various segments of the practice.

On a 1 to 10 scale, with 1 being low and 10 being high, rate the following:

1. I feel that *my* personal level of teamwork is ________.
2. The current level of teamwork for the *doctors* is ________.
3. The current level of teamwork in the *technical department* is ________.
4. The current level of teamwork in the *reception/patient accounts department* is ________.
5. The current level of teamwork in the *marketing department* is ________.
6. The current level of teamwork in the *optical department* is ________.
7. The current level of teamwork in the *surgery center* is ________.
8. The current level of teamwork for our *overall* practice is ________, and I believe we should be striving for an *overall* practice teamwork level of ________.

What do you observe from this second part of the self-assessment? Which areas of the practice have higher or lower levels of teamwork? Do you think it's easier to improve overall teamwork when doctor teamwork is high, but teamwork in other areas is faltering, or the reverse, when the lay staff are great at teamwork, but doctor teamwork is poor?

Part Three

As a final—ideally group—exercise, select two or three weak aspects of your practice's teamwork suggested by your responses to the previous questions. For each of these weak areas, write down specific goals and tactics to achieve them. Here's an example:

No one on our team except the administrator and our partner doctors understand how we're doing as a practice. These insiders get the financial and volume performance data, but everyone else on the team can only guess if it's been a good or poor quarter compared to last year. To improve this, we're going to prepare a quarterly scorecard for the practice, containing five key benchmarks for this year vs last. These benchmarks will be: Total patient visits; total surgical cases; a lay staff efficiency ratio consisting of total payroll hours divided by total patient visits; a doctor efficiency ratio consisting of patient visits per clinic hour worked; and the percentile increase or decrease in our collections. We will share this scorecard with every member of our staff at our quarterly all-hands meetings. Whenever our quarterly scorecard shows progress, we'll think up some creative way to celebrate our improvement as a group.

CHAPTER 24

Create a Staff Team of Engaged "Employee-preneurs"

When employees join executives in truly owning the responsibility for business success, an exciting new sense of teamwork takes hold.
—Punit Renjen

Employees have three prime needs: Interesting work, recognition for doing a good job, and being let in on things that are going on in the company.
—Zig Ziglar

A term that's been kicking around human resource management circles for many years is *intrapreneur*, connoting a worker who, instead of leaving the firm, sticks around and behaves entrepreneurially … digging deeper, working harder, taking initiative and reasonable risks, not only for his or her own benefit, but for the benefit of the company.

Another term for the same behavior, with perhaps a bit more relevance to your practice setting, is being an *employee-preneur*. Here are a few examples:

- The tech who, on his or her own, discovers an opportunity to negotiate for lower supply pricing
- The receptionist who comes to the administrator with an idea to shave staff hours without decreasing customer service

Wohl C, Pinto JB. *UP: Taking Ophthalmic Administrators and Their Management Teams to the Next Level of Skill, Performance, and Career Satisfaction, Second Edition* (pp 131-133).

- The junior biller who runs a report before being asked by management, discovering that some YAGs and special tests are not being posted and submitted for payment
- The associate optometrist who volunteers to investigate the practice's surgical outcomes and compare them to national baselines

These "above and beyond the call" behaviors are something you would expect of practice owners and managers, but not of rank-and-file staff.

It is easy to see how your eye clinic is more likely to be an incubator for employee-preneurs than the average hardware store, corner deli, or factory floor:

- The mission to treat and prevent eye disease is noble and, more often than not, the cure is dramatic, immediate, and enduring.
- There are a limited number of common eye diseases and treatments, so any thoughtful lay staffer with no prior medical knowledge can come pretty quickly to an understanding of the services your practice provides, and from there, spot inefficiencies.
- Doctors are cultural heroes. Digging deep to help your doctor provide better care comes naturally.

Here are six things you can do to encourage employee-preneurism:

1. **Start at the top.** Owners and managers must embrace entrepreneurial thinking if you are going to have any hope encouraging entrepreneurism in line staff. Hold a board-level discussion of what entrepreneurism means in the context of your unique practice. What meanings fit? Risk tolerance? Initiative? Flying in the face of convention? Innovation? An orientation to finding and solving customer wants and needs?
2. **Foster strategic intimacy.** As Zig Ziglar counseled, employees need to be let in on the company's broader mission and status. You don't have to send out boardroom transcripts to accomplish this. At least once per year, you and the managing partner should be updating the practice's strategic plan and key performance indicators. A sanitized version of this can be shared with staff, along the lines of "Smith Eye Care has had a very good year. We were hoping to grow 5% in patient volumes, but achieved 8% growth this year. Over the course of the next 12 months, we don't plan to add or subtract any providers or services, but we will be working hard to increase the practice's cataract volumes to reach the 60 cases per month needed to give us confidence to proceed with our own surgery center. In order to accomplish this, we will be shifting to a full-time surgical counselor, and will be increasing our outreach to optometrists. Each of you can play a role in this by treating our OD-referred patients like VIPs, and we'll be asking for volunteers soon to aid our outreach efforts."

3. **Teach staff how the company works.** In addition to telling staff where your practice is going in the future, let them know what makes it tick. For example, most staff underestimate the cost of running a modern practice. You can drive home the importance of time efficiency and filling every appointment slot by teaching them that "Even though we start seeing our first appointment by 8:30 a.m., we don't cover the cost of staff salaries and benefits until 11:30 a.m., and we don't finish paying for rent and utilities until way after lunchtime. Just missing one patient appointment each day over the course of 1 year costs the practice the equivalent of one staffer's annual salary."
4. **Train, train, train.** Staff who are chronically behind in their job knowledge can hardly be expected to think a few steps ahead and anticipate better ways to do things. The secondary gain from this training will be better support for you each clinic day and a lower staff turnover. Staff who know how to do their jobs generally enjoy their work more and stick around.
5. **Encourage risk. Provide positive feedback.** Create a safe environment for staff to try out ideas. Even the brightest member of your staff may come to you with a dozen naïve or impractical suggestions before coming up with a winner. Every time a staffer comes to you with something that won't work, take the time to gush at his or her initiative and creativity and suggest more fruitful pursuits: "Susan, I'm really impressed that you noticed how convoluted our injectable drug inventory process is after just 3 months on the job. Your idea to streamline the process is something we considered, but it would leave us without the needed checks and balances to ensure we're not losing $2000 vials of medicine. However, I love your creativity in this whole sphere of inventory controls. I'm going to have you meet with our ambulatory surgical center nurse director and see if we can harness some of that creativity with less costly and less critical materials. With thinking like yours, you're going to go far in this field."
6. **Reward employee-preneurs**. This has to go beyond a $25 gift certificate for the best staff idea of the month. Think about the last staff idea you implemented that really paid off (by reducing costs without reducing quality or increasing quality without increasing costs). Put a dollar value on this recent idea. If the practice saved $20,000/year, a $1000 award would be very reasonable. Think up a name for the award (you could name it after a beloved staffer who has retired, a "Molly"). Present the award at your next staff meeting, with the announcement, "Two times a year we are going to be making an award for nonmanagerial staff who make actionable suggestions that improve patient care and practice performance." Even more than money, lavish praise on your employee-preneurs, which can be more motivating to the kind of people who are willing to step up and make recommendations.

CHAPTER 25

Problem Solving and the Benefits (and Limits) of Practice Task Force Committee Work

A camel is a horse designed by committee.
—Alec Issigonis

A committee is a group of people who individually can do nothing, but who, as a group, can meet and decide that nothing can be done.
—Fred Allen

For years, we've urged clients and audiences to adopt a simple, five-step, one-size-fits-all way to address every practice problem:

- Gather in one room the facts and statistics associated with the problem or opportunity. For example, if a provider's schedule consistency runs behind, you might reasonably need:
  ____ A brief history of when the problem started and how it has developed
  ____ The provider's current template
  ____ The results of a time study showing a typical patient's movement though the clinic
  ____ The provider's actual recent morning and afternoon arrival times
  ____ Comments from staff in the trenches

____ Comments from patients about how they feel when the clinic runs late

____ Monthly patient counts for the provider, compared to norms for the number of patients an average peer can reasonably transit

- In the same room, gather the people who touch the problem or opportunity. In the case of the scheduling problem, this might include:

  ____ The affected provider

  ____ The provider's lead technician

  ____ The department heads of reception and technical services

  ____ The practice administrator (at least in smaller practices)
- Discuss the problem, considering both the facts on the surface ("Dr. Smith's clinics run 60 minutes late throughout the day") and the less-obvious, sometimes-uncomfortable root causes ("Dr. Smith routinely arrives in the office at 9:15 a.m. for his first 8:00 a.m. patient").
- Unless you have solved the problem on the spot, nominate someone who is going to take charge of a new, brief-lived, problem-focused task force, and ask, "What's your deadline for coming up with an actionable solution and solving this problem?"
- Then let your task force do its work and hold the leader responsible for nailing the self-imposed deadline.

This approach comes as close to a universal multitool solution as anything we have in the business of ophthalmology.

This five-step universal solution is so simple, why isn't it used more often? First, because committee work is so often mocked, and second, because of the exceptional culture of medicine. Surgeons are trained to think and act more on their own than collaboratively. This ethos seeps through practices and results in a culture of, "Go figure it out for yourself."

We've dropped into many practices where individuals have puzzled for months over a problem that subsequently yielded quickly to groupthink.

Some practices get halfway to collaboration, but fall short. A problem may be brainstormed in the tech department, but without the input of other team members from billing or marketing or the call center. Break down the silos in your practice and ask, "Who else contributes to this problem? Who else will be affected by our solution?"

By creating successive, brief, interdisciplinary working groups, you not only solve problems faster, you also:

- Break down the barriers that commonly result in techs saying, "The front desk goofs off while we're dying back here" (and vice versa!).
- Build teamwork by allowing staff who would not ordinarily rub shoulders to work together.
- Encourage cross-training and career mobility, as everyone is eventually exposed to every area of the practice.
- Achieve greater buy-in with difficult but necessary decisions.
- Improve morale by giving a wider voice to staff ideas.
- Develop leadership skills by passing the baton to different "problem owners."

- Find out faster if the agreed-upon solution is working because several people will be watching for positive results.
- Take pressure off the managing partner and administrator, leaving them to deal with larger problems by delegating to special, focused committees.

Try to avoid these common missteps in your targeted committee work:

- Get your organizational basics in order. A diverse group of problem solvers will better serve their practice if you have hardwired your practice's culture and general mission.
- Don't use task forces to replace leadership. If an obvious course of action is indicated, proceed rather than losing time to committee work. As the old maxim goes (with apologies to our herpetological readers), "When you see a snake, kill a snake; don't form a snake committee."
- Such focused teams are not the same as standing committees. They should be disbanded as soon as the problem is solved, and not linger.
- Some of the most effective, creative people do their best thinking alone. Feel free to empower a committee-of-one in circumstances where an interdisciplinary approach is not critical.
- Try not to call on the same people time after time when problems surface. Mix it up, encourage the involvement of staff wallflowers.
- Supply adequate resources. If your task force has to meet before or after hours, pay overtime to nonexempt staffers.
- Keep your task forces as small as possible to get the job done. Don't draft five members if two or three will do. As quoted in *The Economist*, Amazon's founder Jeff Bezos once quipped, "If I see more than two pizzas for lunch, I know the team is too big."

• • •

Note that, seen positively, this all-in-one solution works as well for opportunities as it does for problems. Perhaps you've seen this common boardroom phenomenon: Someone will mention a new opportunity, it could be an office to open, a doctor to hire, or a new piece of capital equipment to buy. Lively discussion ensues, and without disciplined chairmanship, can go on for 20 minutes, until someone changes the topic and everyone goes off in a new direction, with no closure on the opportunity raised. When new ideas surface that deserve company attention, the effective chair delegates to a colleague the task of leading a work group to come back to the boardroom with recommendations.

Section V

People Are at the Heart of Our Job

Human Resources Management

CHAPTER 26

Fifteen Tips to Avoid Bad Practice Hires

Hiring people is like making friends. Pick good ones, and they'll enrich your life. Make bad choices, and they'll bring you down.
—Jason Fried

Often the best solution to a management problem is the right person.
—Edwin Booz

You can have the best strategy and the best building in the world, but if you don't have the hearts and minds of the people who work with you, none of it comes to life.
—Renee West

Bad hires hurt all over. First, they waste your time and money being recruited. Then they work slowly, make expensive mistakes, and bring down the morale of fellow staffers. Finally, it costs money and time to replace them. As if that wasn't enough, your self-confidence as an administrator takes a beating.

Every practice we know has at least one proverbial bad apple in the barrel, and even the smartest administrators and practice owners make dozens of hiring goofs in the course of a career. It comes with the territory.

You don't have to become a hiring genius to materially improve in this area. Small wins count big. Just consider baseball's common metric: batting average.

Wohl C, Pinto JB. *UP: Taking Ophthalmic Administrators and Their Management Teams to the Next Level of Skill, Performance, and Career Satisfaction, Second Edition* (pp 141-143).

Hitting the ball just 4 out of 10 times at bat is exceptional performance. Babe Ruth had a lifetime average of hitting the ball 3.42 times for every 10 times at bat. Hitting it 3 times is about average. If you only hit it 2 times, they'll kick you off the team.

Hiring the right people at every level within your practice is critical to creating and maintaining successful operations, profitability, and brand integrity.

Here are some tips for selecting top talent, people who can bring more value and be a better fit with your culture.

1. Always hire with a clear, updated, written description of the job. This forces everyone inside the practice to get quite literally on the same page about the needed skills.
2. Ask: "Do we really need to hire?" Most practices in the United States are modestly overstaffed. Don't just replace a departing worker by rote … ask yourself if there's another option (eg, shifting duties to others, streamlining office procedures, paying overtime here or there, bringing in seasonal workers). You'll never have to fire the person you don't hire.
3. If you are replacing a departing member of your staff with whom you are on good terms, have him or her interview your finalists … nobody knows the job better than the last person doing it.
4. As Jim Collins wrote in his classic book, *Good to Great*, "Hire first for character, then for technical skills." This is difficult to accomplish in the space of a brief interview. Expand the time spent with final candidates by having two interviews on separate days or arranging a half-day to job-shadow. Are they punctual? Do they show an interest in those around them or seem self-absorbed? Are they patient and focused when you describe the job?
5. Ask this character-challenging question, "Tell me about a time when you made a very big and perhaps costly mistake during your career, how it played out, and what you learned from this experience." More mature candidates will always take personal responsibility for their mistakes, humbly acknowledge any wrongdoing, and be able to report growth as a result of bouncing back from the error of their ways. By contrast, less mature, even dysfunctional, individuals will more likely make excuses, blame others, and shirk responsibility for previous work-related problems, and, as a result, be unable to describe any valuable lesson learned.
6. It's a gross simplification to be sure, but there are really only two kinds of people in the world: givers and takers. We all have a pretty well-honed intuition, often within a few minutes of meeting someone new, in which category they fit. Hire only givers.
7. Everyone who interacts with your patients must have a "heart for service"—a genuine interest in and heartfelt desire for helping people, including both teammates and patients. Screen for candidates with prior experience helping others (this could be a formal job or volunteer work). Ask your candidate, "As someone applying for a job where we are helping patients—often frail older adults—what can you tell me about your background and interest in serving others?"

8. Ask job applicants, "Tell me about your first paying job." Our experience over a combined 75 years in the field has shown us that the best workers we encounter in our consulting work—both doctors and lay staff—started their work life very early as baby sitters, paper carriers, lawn mowers, sidewalk shovelers, and the like.
9. Especially for more critical hires (eg, doctors, managers) always arrange a working interview. Such an interview takes place over the course of a regular workday, meeting with and shadowing various staff, and sharing a couple of meals with selected members of the team.
10. To the extent possible, apply these and other practical tests to final candidates:
    - Watch a senior tech candidate work up a staff member.
    - Give a biller candidate a few charts to code and ask them to place a mock collection call.
    - Ask a receptionist to answer a mock phone call from you (and you should pretend to be a difficult patient).
    - You can even give a practical test to trainee candidates. Have a tech/scribe candidate demonstrate memory skills by reciting back a long, compound sentence. To test for dexterity, use the simple children's game of pick-up-sticks (keep a box of toothpicks in the office).
11. If you are hiring a provider, always have a doctor from your practice travel to the candidate's current clinical setting to watch the candidate in action. Never hire a surgeon, especially a partner-track doctor, who has not been personally observed in the operating room by a physician representative of your practice. (You are not just looking for surgical skills but how a prospective provider performs globally during the most stressful part of a surgeon's life. Watching interactions with the operating room staff tells volumes.)
12. Listen to the reasonable objections and doubts expressed by current staff about a candidate. They will be looking at a candidate from a different perspective than your own. But realize that some of their hesitation may be motivated more by jealousy or fear of being shown up, than by what's in the company's best interests.
13. Don't settle. Make sure your candidate pool is large enough to increase the odds of finding someone who is just right for the position. Always ask yourself or the search committee, "Will our team be weaker, the same, or stronger if this person joins us?"
14. If relocation will be required for a new provider or senior-level manager, consider the candidate's spouse/partner/family. Ensure that there are practical cultural, spouse employment, recreational, religious, and educational fits. A significant percentage of partner-track surgeons leave before making partner simply because their spouses are unhappy.
15. The most important candidate characteristic for bringing value to your practice is an eagerness to support a mission and purpose greater than oneself, indicated by an unselfish work ethic, supportive team spirit, and previous activities (often unpaid) in support of mission work or other social causes. By contrast, candidates who seem to be self-absorbed, entitled, and otherwise showing an inflated sense of self-importance are more likely to demonstrate a self-centered focus rather than team spirit once on your payroll, stirring up drama and strife, and eroding team spirit.

CHAPTER 27

Optimizing Staff Training

I hated every minute of training, but I said, don't quit. Suffer now and live the rest of your life as a champion.
—Muhammad Ali

If you are doing something the same way you have been doing it for 10 years; the chances are you are doing it wrong.
—Charles F. Kettering

Physicians in training learn early the boiled-down, three-step medical training rubric "See one, do one, teach one." But this simplistic mantra, while adequate for über-smart and motivated students in medical school, is insufficient guidance in today's ophthalmic practice setting.

While every fortunate practice has a few lay staff stars, it is unlikely that your practice's entire support staff can learn at the same pace your doctors probably did. Nor do you necessarily want to hire a receptionist or technician who is so whip-smart that they'll learn their job in a week and be leaving your practice for graduate school in year. It's tempting but not practical for the long run.

Wohl C, Pinto JB. *UP: Taking Ophthalmic Administrators and Their Management Teams to the Next Level of Skill, Performance, and Career Satisfaction, Second Edition* (pp 145-149). © 2021 Taylor & Francis Group.

Indeed, if you reflect on your own practice setting, some of the most competent and valued support staff you employ probably took a bit longer to learn their job than you would have wished. But today, they perform their routine tasks flawlessly. And they do so without the boredom that sets in when you hire staff who will ultimately be drawn away to a role other than health care patient services.

As an intense, smart administrator yourself, it's easy to fall into the habit of hiring smart, ambitious people like you and letting them organically figure out how to do their job (sometimes diverging from what's efficient or best for patient care), rather than hiring less-costly, often longer-tenured, happy-to-work-in-the-same-job-same-place workers and training them to do everything your way ... every time ... for years.

Better training is at the heart of this approach. If you create systems that can reliably teach a motivated, pleasant, but less experienced individual from off the street any nonsupervisory job in your office within 6 months, you'll be a more effective business manager and more confident in your control over operations. You'll also stop being held hostage by one staffer or another whom you "couldn't possibly lose."

"How to train" is an important enough subject in eye care that it's worth stopping for a moment and reflecting on how you train today and improvements you can make. And it is just as important, perhaps more so, to review how you are training your practice's trainers.

Success Factors

Like surgery, the intended outcomes in business are foremost. We want to launch any business initiative with the ending clearly in mind. The more specific the outcome is set and communicated, the better. This operates at two levels, one wide and one narrow. Both should be easy for you to articulate based on the overall goals you have for the practice.

Your wide goals for better training might include:

- Lower costs by hiring inexperienced staff rather than high-cost veterans (although some practices do choose to hire highly experienced staff and then expect more productivity from each to offset the increased costs associated with this tactic)
- Achieving a higher level of support staff mastery on the floor, and doing it faster, so the doctors are freed up to see more patients
- Speeding up patient throughput in all practice stations, from the front desk to optical
- Being more attractive to less experienced job candidates
- Improving staff tenure with better training (staffers who know their jobs well are usually happier and less likely to leave)

And here are some examples of narrow goals for training:

- Reduce the tech work-up component of the average examination from 25 minutes to 18 by teaching techs how to eliminate unnecessary history questions
- Reduce front desk demographics posting errors from 10% to 2% or less by reinforcing the importance of double-checking all entries
- Elevate the net collection ratio (percent of allowable charges collected) from 90% to 95% or higher with a billing department tune-up

Both the broad and narrow goals should be clear, spelled out in writing, and shared with the team before you launch a formal training or retraining initiative.

Of course, to be successful with any new training initiative, your practice's underlying teamwork has to be good or better. Teamwork and high staff morale provide the motivation to teach and learn, as well as the group cohesion to want to help everyone on the team achieve a given level of competency. Better-trained staff will tend to be more satisfied teammates, and vice versa.

Cross-training throughout the practice is critical. You should train everyone generally, and individuals specifically. Here's an example from a completely different field:

On a NASCAR pit crew, just one person is ordinarily assigned the job of jacking up the car so the tires can be changed. But everyone can handle the job. In NASCAR, one teammate's minor error can lose the race (sound familiar)? So the specialized training regimen is obsessive. According to *Circle Track Magazine*, a trade publication, one training method many teams use involves a cardboard mock-up of a racing tire and a marker pen. While on his knees, the tire changer takes the marker and touches it to the dummy lug nuts in the pattern he needs to use with the air gun, just as fast as he possibly can.

This reinforces the pattern, improves concentration and gives the tire changer a significant amount of muscle memory for the next full-bore pit stop. Imagine what the same training diligence would do to shave seconds off the time it takes your tech to get a Tono-Pen (Reichert, Inc) reading.

It's important that you understand the baseline skills of your current workers. It's not uncommon for us to see a doctor presenting an advanced didactic, theoretical lecture to the technicians, when what they really need is hands-on basic training. It's best to not impose an uninformed syllabus on a workgroup, but rather, ask them and their direct supervisor what skills would be the most helpful to transfer. This week. This month. This year.

Are you setting aside enough time for training? As general guidance, we tell clients that they should provide about 1 hour of formal training time for every 80 hours (2 weeks) worked.

Try wherever possible to provide a practice-based context for what you are trying to teach, in a way that touches the staff directly. Here's an example: "We're going to be shifting our refraction fee from $40 to $47. We are doing this because it will put us in line with our colleagues in the area. We know that this may seem to be a big leap to you, but it has been 5 years since our last increase. And if it helps, consider this: the extra $7 we will now charge will pay for one person's salary here in our practice. Think of that the next time you feel shy about asking patients to pay their refraction fee at check-out."

How do you currently reward staff for completion of each training cycle? This reward need not, in most settings, be a permanent advancement in title or pay, but rather some tangible, public recognition: a pin on the staff member's name tag; a letter of recognition signed off by the owners, or a shout-out in the biweekly staff newsletter. Of course, reaching significant training hallmarks should come with more than a pat on the back. Many practices find it helpful to fractionate staffing levels (eg, Tech Level II, Billing Level 1) and to kick payroll ranges up a notch when a higher threshold is met.

Plan ahead. Rather than springing a training session on staff at the last minute, schedule these sessions in advance throughout the year. Reduce anxiety. Let staff know what each training session will involve.

Train the trainers. Be sure to train billing supervisors, front desk leads, and head techs before you set them out to train their staff.

Assist your supervisors. Help them supply readings and self-assessments to their staff several days before you start a training session. This will prepare the staff for what's coming, as well as save time on routine information, get all the students up to speed on the same basics, and set the right tone for your supervisor's role in a given training module.

Finally, there is little business purpose in overtraining, or paying people for learning skills that are not directly relevant to their current position. Every practice needs a certain number of junior level, certified ophthalmic assistants, or lower techs, because not all jobs require high-level skills. It's unnecessary, at least in dry business terms and financial perspective, to insist that all of your technicians gain certified ophthalmic technician designation, or that every tech learn to be a surgical scrub.

Leading practices strive to be learning organizations, where staff training is a priority and physician-owners give their own time and considerable resources to bring new staff up to speed and continuously improve the skills of experienced staff. Here's a self-assessment to complete as a group exercise to measure selected dimensions of your practice's training and education efforts. This list of attributes is by no means complete, and no practice could be expected to have high scores in all these areas. Feel free to add any dimensions of better training that you think are important in your practice.

Training and Education Assessment Scorecard

Score each item on this 20-point list based on the following scale:

5 = I strongly agree with this statement.

4 = I agree with this statement.

3 = I am neutral; I neither agree or disagree with this statement.

2 = I disagree with this statement.

1 = I strongly disagree with this statement.

_____ 1. Our policy and procedure manuals are complete and up to date for each department.

_____ 2. These policy and procedure manuals are used as active training documents, not just kept on a shelf.

_____ 3. We use a formal onboarding checklist for each new staffer to ensure each is well oriented.

_____ 4. We arrange at least 2 formal hours of ongoing training per experienced support staffer per month.

_____ 5. The providers are all on the same page; techs just have to memorize one agreed-upon protocol, not many.

_____ 6. We cross-train staff, work-up techs know how to scribe, check-in clerks know how to check out.

_____ 7. Our working managers personally know how to do each job they supervise.

_____ 8. Staff turnover is low, so we don't unduly lose the staff we train.

_____ 9. Managers and doctors in our practice personally demonstrate patience when they teach.

_____ 10. Each department has at least one formally designated, effective trainer.

_____ 11. We keep track of who has learned what, so we have a clear roadmap for continuing education.

_____ 12. In addition to written training materials, we use video clips to help reinforce skills development.

_____ 13. Our training content strikes the right balance between theory and practical how-to knowledge.

_____ 14. Our training accommodates different learning styles and especially includes a lot of hands-on activity.

_____ 15. We use excellent training materials and visual learning aids.

_____ 16. We realize that everyone learns at their own pace, and we provide repetition for slower learners.

_____ 17. Our training sessions are kept interesting and lively, they are not dull lectures.

_____ 18. Staffers in every department are formally recredentialed at least annually.

_____ 19. We visit other practices and go to conferences to learn how to do things better

_____ 20. Our doctors train as seriously as staff, attending conferences and keeping up their continuing education credits and skills.

Total Score: _________

Add up your score. With 20 different attributes, and with up to 5 points each, there's a maximum score of 100. This summary score can be a valuable internal baseline of your educational efforts and can help point out areas to improve. It might be interesting to repeat this scoring instrument again in 6 months or 1 year. As a final—ideally group—exercise, select two or three weaker aspects of your practice's educational and training efforts that are suggested by your responses to the questions. For each of these weak areas, write down specific goals, tactics to achieve them, and deadlines.

CHAPTER 28

Motivating Your Practice Staff

Those who try to do something and fail are infinitely better than those who try to do nothing and succeed.
—Lloyd Jones

Be who you are and say what you feel because those who mind don't matter and those who matter don't mind.
—Dr. Seuss

If you do not treat people with the respect they deserve, do not expect any kind of commitment to your productivity goals and target.
—Ian Fuhr

You are the boss. But mere bossiness is not enough. The most effective administrators have finessed the skill of getting other people to want to do things for them. This is the distinguishing factor between being a manager vs being a leader ... being an inspiration to others.

While your original training may be in accounting or marketing or medicine, the most important daily skills you must bring to the job as administrator or manager need to be much broader, and often very intuitive. You must be able to motivate talent, improving the weakest half of your people while vigorously rewarding the strongest half. You have to be a coach rather than a criticizer, molding the ever-shifting, fragile human ingredients to ultimately better serve your patients.

Wohl C, Pinto JB. *UP: Taking Ophthalmic Administrators and Their Management Teams to the Next Level of Skill, Performance, and Career Satisfaction, Second Edition* (pp 151-154).

In truth, just how your practice turns out each day depends largely on how well you can do all of this. It counts for much more than your objective accounting, marketing, or clinical skills.

It's easy to coach a tech to take a more accurate intraocular pressure reading. But can you as readily coach that staffer to be more interested career-wise? To be more thoughtful in handling expensive instruments? To be kinder to patients and fellow workers?

While spring-loaded, self-motivated staff can sometimes be selected during the hiring process, most performance, in most practices, is, at least at the outset, externally launched by effective physician and lay leadership. But let's assume you already have a pretty great team. What can you do to get the most from it? After many years of watching some of the most talented managers and business owners at work, here are some of the top skills they apply.

First and foremost, great practice managers are constantly improving themselves. To do this, you must do more than simply read the business literature or attend national meetings. You need to start by not being defensive. Sharp managers readily accept constructive, even negative, feedback from team members.

Doing so is self-reinforcing. When you say, "You know, you may be right, tell me more" even to the most hypercritical staffer you supervise, you'll start getting feedback that's faster, more useful, and more honest.

In order to obtain this feedback, you can't be talking all the time. You have to listen. This is sometimes easier to do one-on-one than during group sessions, such as department meetings, where your staff are looking to you for all the answers. Be sure to build into every group meeting a formal time for brainstorming and going around the table for input.

People have long memories of how you make them feel. And most workers are pretty good about picking up on your opinion of their talents and will perform accordingly. If you're sending signals that say, "I think you're going to blow this assignment," chances are a worker will live down to your expectations. So no matter how many times a staff member has disappointed you, assume that he or she has hidden talents that you have just not been able to bring out yet.

This can yield surprising results. The next time you hand out an assignment to someone you're on the fence about, try this. Accompany your request with the statement, "Mary, in the past I think I've unfairly misjudged your abilities. I know you can do this project. In fact, I'm sure of it. Let's start with a clean slate for you here at our eye center."

Try to not be the kind of boss who supplies all of the answers. Even though you're probably the smartest and hardest working member of your team, leave some room for creativity by the staff you manage. People like having control and are more motivated when they enjoy the satisfaction of solving their own problems.

When giving feedback and handing out assignments, especially to a newer member of your staff, try being a little more "suggestive" and a little less "directive." By being just a little too directive, especially with people you have not yet learned to read, you can bring out a defensive response that will take weeks or even years to overcome.

Always emphasize the positive. When you catch your staff doing things right encourage them to continue such achievement, rather than dwelling on what's been done wrong. This positive approach is often difficult for managers and doctors who hold themselves to high expectations—and give themselves a healthy daily dose of negative criticism. The same negativity you apply to yourself just naturally spills out to others. While you may think this will evoke the desired improvement in performance, the opposite is actually the case. Most employees will simply shut down under negative reinforcement, shrinking from trying to learn new skills and missing opportunities to improve by taking on duties that are at the edge of their competency.

Fearless, fair, and well-timed confrontation is a critical administrative coaching skill. Even while remaining positive, it's important to call attention to performance gaps and not sweep important behavioral gaffs or technical errors under the rug. Every great manager must find an individual balance in this area.

The tipping point between tough and fair is decidedly not static. Every worker changes over the course of a career, and your threshold and timing for bringing things up has to be flexible. On top of this, your own skills and perceptions change over time. Knowing when to apply the correct, nuanced pressure in the right areas separates exceptional managers from those who lose nearly as many points as they gain with their staff and boards over time.

In most practices, administrators and managers spend nearly as much administrative time directing doctors as they do leading lay staff. Although it can be difficult, especially for a younger manager, work on being as comfortable confronting these nominal superiors as you are confronting your own staff. Most doctors, especially those who tend to be insecure and bullying, have far more respect for their managers who are fearless and stand their ground on difficult issues.

Context is critical whether you are addressing problems or opportunities. Before describing a performance deficit or a desired new goal with a member of your staff, make sure that you both agree on the person's strengths and weaknesses of past performance. Then, make sure the staffer understands the rewards of being able to reach a new standard or goal; you like rewards and so do your staff. At the end of a coaching moment, make sure you have your colleague's commitment. When appropriate, put the agreement in writing and even have staff sign a formal commitment to major initiatives.

Remember that most of us like to feel we are part of something larger than ourselves. Make it a point during group meetings to discuss the history of your practice and the leaps you have made since then. Let people know as specifically as you can how they have been a part of your success as an organization.

People are motivated by role models. Look at the influence that motivational experts (Dale Carnegie, Tony Robbins, and the like) have had on the world. If you don't think you are a particularly motivating person, read books and listen to recordings and podcasts from speakers like these. Adopt their tone, their concepts, and their energy and you'll not only better motivate your staff, you'll also be personally better motivated.

Finally, realize that your coaching style may not fit the needs of every worker. Your challenge is to recognize what does and does not work with each member of your staff and learn to modify your approach to get the best work from all of them. With experience, however, you'll pick workers who not only perform their core job functions well but will also be responsive to your particular approach to supervision.

CHAPTER 29

Recognizing Staff Contributions to Your Practice

Nothing else can quite substitute for a few well-chosen, well-timed, sincere words of praise. They're absolutely free and worth a fortune.
—Sam Walton

Give thanks for a little and you will find a lot.
—Hansa proverb

It's often the small things in life that count most to your staff and resonate within them when the external noise of clinic life recedes. No matter what their roles are in the organization, they want to be recognized for strong efforts and contributions. It is human nature to want to be acknowledged.

The recognition need not be monumental. A "thank you" at the end of a tough clinic day, a lunch celebration for a successful group effort that met an operational goal, or a special shout-out at the all-hands staff meeting for an achievement all accomplish more than you may imagine.

Wohl C, Pinto JB. *UP: Taking Ophthalmic Administrators and Their Management Teams to the Next Level of Skill, Performance, and Career Satisfaction, Second Edition* (pp 155-158).

Recognition is most effective when it is timely and customized to the individual. For example, a grandstanding, bold staff member will love to hear your praise at a staff meeting, but the same public acknowledgment for an extremely introverted employee may not be motivational in the same way.

Luckily, you have a nearly infinite number of ways to praise your team.

Why are recognition and appreciation important parts of practice management? Shouldn't employees just do their jobs because they are paid to do so? Research shows that the number one reason people leave their jobs is lack of recognition for their efforts. Income ranks fourth on that same list. So, even if you cynically feel that a paycheck should be enough, it's in your best interest as the practice administrator or department head to learn how to recognize staff performance effectively.

As we continue to move through generally uncertain economic times, which will continue to drive reimbursement reductions to ophthalmology specifically, labor costs will grow, requiring focused attention and control. This includes core wages and benefits, employee retention, and recruitment and training costs.

Just as it is more cost effective to retain a patient than recruit a new one, the same applies to staffing for your practice. Small, inexpensive staff recognition efforts that boost staff tenure can forestall costly recruiting costs.

Does praising and recognizing staff come naturally? Not in all organizations, and certainly not in ophthalmology, a setting where many surgeons famously don't speak up until they are disappointed by staff performance.

Recognizing and appreciating staff should be an obvious business habit and come naturally to your management team members, since most of us like to be treated that way ourselves. And yet, staff recognition is often applied intermittently or skipped altogether, even in otherwise great organizations.

Here are a few things to consider about employee recognition and how to implement a consistent commitment to this important process in your practice.

Acknowledge the importance of a consistent practice philosophy to support employee recognition:

- Teach your board and front-line managers that recognition is a powerful tool. It can result in improved employee engagement, increased productivity, greater creativity, and more loyalty to the practices' success.
- Send the message to your staff that the physician board, you as administrator, and department managers are all involved and supportive of the process. If it is perceived that the doctors are not supporting senior management or that you don't prioritize it like the department managers, a critical piece of the puzzle will be missing.
- Provide training and education to your managers so it becomes part of your practice culture.
- Designate a departmental budget line for staff recognition activities, if appropriate in your setting.

Some managers do not use recognition as a tool because they:

- Are unsure how to best recognize staff.
- Don't perceive it as a priority and use lack of time as an excuse.
- Feel that previous recognition efforts have not been appreciated or have evolved into entitlements.
- Think that the organization as a whole doesn't support this effort, so implementation becomes a burden on the departmental level.

Examples of the most appreciated and effective types of recognition include:

- Physician and managerial acknowledgment of accomplishments both small and large. This could range from a stellar clinic day accomplished with short staffing, up to meeting all Merit-based Incentive Payment System criteria for a specific time period.
- Praise in the form of handwritten notes, emails, or public mention.
- Catching an employee doing the right thing, a bit above and beyond, and being recognized the same day with a small gift card for lunch or movie tickets.
- Formal programs, such as length of service awards, employee referral bonuses, implementable suggestions rewards, etc.
- Tapping into the American Academy of Ophthalmic Executives Listserv as a great way to find and share ideas with your peers.

Evaluate the success of your efforts:

- Perform employee satisfaction surveys at least annually basis. Poll your employees in a nonthreatening, informal way to assess their feelings about being appreciated in your organization (see the sample survey format in Chapter 30).
- Be sure to ask for feedback about the practice's employee recognition efforts in detail during employee exit interviews. There is generally no better way to get the real scoop from a staffer than when there is no fear of retribution if the exiting employee doesn't agree with you.
- Don't be surprised if staff recognition is perceived to be significantly different between departments, even if you have a practice-wide policy. Because we are talking about human behavior and perception, on both sides (employees and managers), this is a common finding.

Review the results of collected feedback at your regularly held managers' meetings:

- As a learning opportunity during management team meetings, require that specific, appropriate examples of adverse conduct by staffers be discussed openly by your managers so that everyone can learn from the situation, not just the affected department head. It is common for us to hear from newer managers that they are stumped in the human resources (HR) area and learn a lot when they hear how their more-experienced peers handle HR challenges.
- Identify the stars in your practice who shine in this area. Have those managers and doctors mentor the rest of the management team, aiming for practice-wide consistency and incremental improvements.

Success with your staff recognition efforts enhances the likelihood of your employees repeatedly doing good work. When your employees feel generally appreciated and even especially noticed for extra effort, they in turn pass along the positive notes to co-workers and patients.

Keeping the rewards fresh, relevant, personalized, and contingent on a desired behavior or performance will result in all parties valuing the outcome. And, as financial resources to support escalating expenses continue to taper, nonfinancial or low-cost tools become more critical adjuncts to successful practice management.

CHAPTER 30

Avoiding the High Cost of Staff Turnover Rates

Quitting is the easiest thing to do.
—Robert Kiyosaki

While determination builds character,
quitting is habit forming.
—Frank Sonnenberg

Wisdom stems from personality accountability.
We all make mistakes; own them ... learn from them.
Don't throw away the lesson by blaming others.
—Steve Maraboli

Typical adult workers in the United States have been at their present job about 4 years. That's in line with the typical turnover rate among lay support staff in ophthalmology today.

Expressed in different units, that's about a 25% turnover rate—the percent of staffers who leave each year for any reason.

Some manufacturers have a 10% turnover rate, Amazon has a roughly 100% turnover rate, and turnover rates in fast food can approach 200%. Of course, it only takes a few hours to learn your job as a new line cook at McDonald's or a few days to learn how to be a new warehouse worker at Amazon, so high turnover rates there are less disruptive, but it's very problematic in an ophthalmology clinic, where it can take years to learn how to be a highly competent technician or biller.

Wohl C, Pinto JB. *UP: Taking Ophthalmic Administrators and Their Management Teams to the Next Level of Skill, Performance, and Career Satisfaction, Second Edition* (pp 159-161).

Although eye care's 25% turnover rate is what we see most commonly in our consulting work, we also see stressed practices with more than 50% rates—and a few practices with 10% rates and lower.

Here are eight fast tips for increasing staff tenure:

1. Measure your turnover rate. Divide the number of lay staffers who left your practice (for any reason) in the last 12 months, by the total number of workers you typically employ. If you lost 5 staff and employ 20, that's a 25% turnover rate—roughly the average in our field. Be concerned if it's over 30%. Be alarmed at 50% or higher.
2. Measure staff morale. This can be as easy as a brief, three-question, confidential survey:

Please rate staff morale on a 0 to 10 scale where 0 is low/terrible, 10 is high/wonderful:

In the past few weeks, staff morale has been:	
About 6 months ago, staff morale was:	
About 1 year ago, staff morale was:	

Expand, if you like, with a follow-up question:

Two things we should do this year to build a better practice and improve morale are:

A. ______________________________

B. ______________________________

The collated results of this simple survey will be revealing. We've applied this survey to tens of thousands of staffers over the years; the average morale score is a 6, even in practices with quite-acceptable turnover rates. Average scores above 7 are unusual, but when present, correlate with lower turnover rates. Average scores below 5 are very, very rare, but definitely correlate with higher turnover.

3. Boost workplace enjoyment. People work for love and money, so even if you pay at market rates, you have to provide lots of attentive care. Indeed, there are practices that are forced to pay well below market rates that also have a low turnover rate because administrators and practice owners deeply engage with staff. At the same time, you boost enjoyment, boost staffer-to-staffer connections; one of the greatest determinants of job satisfaction is the relationship we have with our co-workers. Do this with everything from short-term, interdepartmental problem-solving task forces to TGIF gatherings at the end of the week.
4. Have a buddy system for new hires. Every new worker joining your team should be bonded formally for an initial 90-day period to a colleague. This buddy is in addition to the direct supervisor and is usually a peer in the same department. After 90 days, the new staffer will have made connections and found his or her own way in the practice, but this formal approach ensures everyone has at least one friendly face in the practice at the outset.

5. Think of every job as a career. If you don't treat every job in your practice as important, you won't convey a vital message to every worker: "What you do here counts." One of the lowest turnover rates we've seen was in a practice where the solo doctor made it a part of his routine to stop by the records clerk at some point every day to say hello and give thanks. It costs nothing and will keep people bonded to you and the practice.
6. Foster career mastery. Every worker, from surgeons to scrub techs, tends to enjoy work at which they have become a master. Don't let this mastery be an accident in your practice. Foster skills development with a written syllabus of skills to learn for each position, and back this up with formal training time and periodic skills assessments.
7. Provide abundant feedback and accentuate the positive. This is much more than the traditional annual review (see Chapter 36 for employee recognition suggestions). Many surgeons, and by extension their managers, provide negative feedback when an error is detected but no feedback when work is performed at or above par. This is a recipe for low morale. When you find your people doing things right, point it out often and publicly. Make sure this positive feedback is widely distributed, so that every staffer gets your message, "I admire and appreciate the work you do here."
8. Scan for burnout. Very few disaffected staff leave their practices without advance signs of their unhappiness. The administrator, managing partner, and each department head should be on the hunt for these signs: higher absenteeism, late arrival, spending lunchtime alone, and a generally dejected affect. If you want such staffers to leave, by all means accelerate them toward the door. But if you sense that a good worker is a flight risk, address your concerns directly. "It seems you're not as happy in your work here as you once were, which really upsets me because you're such a valuable part of our practice. Can we talk about it?"

Is a very low turnover rate always better? No. Although you may pride yourself on a single-digit turnover rate, this can be a sign that you are too lenient, allowing weak or underperforming staff to overstay. Just like human physiology, balance is the key. Too much or too little insulin can be fatal. Too low a turnover rate may signal a need to set higher standards.

CHAPTER 31

When Is the Right Time to Terminate an Employee?

Trust your gut feeling about things, listen to what others are saying, and look at the results of your actions. Once you know the truth, you can set about taking action to improve. Everyone will be better for it.
—Jack Canfield

Perfectionism and procrastination have such a fine line. You say, "Well, I want it to be good. I want it to be perfect." But what you're really doing is not doing your work. You're putting off showing up and being visible because then you're going to be judged, and it might suck.
—Jen Sincero

Procrastination makes easy things hard, hard things harder.
—Mason Cooley

During a recent presentation, we asked the audience, "How many of you continue to employ at least one person who should have already been dismissed from your practice?" Almost every hand was in the air.

We don't believe that ophthalmic practices have low standards. It's often quite the opposite. But these underperforming or corrosive staff members manage

Wohl C, Pinto JB. *UP: Taking Ophthalmic Administrators and Their Management Teams to the Next Level of Skill, Performance, and Career Satisfaction, Second Edition* (pp 163-167).

to stay employed, often for many years beyond reason, to the chagrin of their most efficient and well-mannered co-workers.

Here are specific tools to help determine when an employee is on track or has finally crossed the line, and how to proceed with employment termination.

Position Descriptions

Every job in the practice needs a written position description that specifies detailed job duties and expected performance.

Position descriptions are best utilized when reviewed and revised annually by the immediate supervisor of the position. When you keep them updated, they are always ready to be used for interviewing potential new hires, as well as being a good reference document for evaluating current employee performance.

Unfortunately, it is common to find these documents filed in a binder, terribly outdated. As with all practice management tools, documents that collect dust on a shelf for years result in missed opportunities for practice improvement.

Annual Performance Reviews

Feedback to employees about their performance supports individual professional growth and organizational alignment. As an administrator or department head, one of your core responsibilities is to foster communication about the goals and expectations you have for every person who works under you. Annual or semiannual performance reviews are key to this responsibility. Reviews should include:

1. Recognition for outstanding work. Make this as specific as you can. Not, "I appreciate you being punctual every morning," but "I appreciate that you get here 10 minutes before your shift, settle in, have a few laughs with your co-workers, and are on the clinic floor starting your first patient at the top of the hour."
2. Acknowledgment of progress made following the guidance that was provided to the employee since the last formal appraisal.
3. Being clear and specific about new opportunities for improvement. You should try to convey a minimum of three <u>measurable</u> goals for the upcoming year. For example, it's clearer to the employee and easier for the manager to determine future success if the goal you state is to "improve patient work-up efficiency by three more patients each day," rather than to simply say, "Work up more patients daily."

Schedule your annual performance review intervals to coincide with each employee's hire date. Practices that perform all the reviews at the same time for all employees find that it encourages salary increase comparisons, staff anxiety, and even an unhelpful "us vs them" mentality, because it's on everyone's mind at the same time. If your current policy is to have all reviews happen at the same time each year, phase this out and shift to anniversary dates.

Practice Standards

Whether you are the office manager of a solo surgeon, who probably conducts performance evaluations alongside you, or the administrator of a larger group working with a deeper management team, it is important to dedicate at least one day each year to review, with the doctor, your aligned organizational goals and performance standards. This exercise can help long term by guiding hiring and firing practices that ultimately lead the practice team you have. Sometimes this is best expressed in terms of the formal values of your practice. Here are examples of representative values that have been adopted at client practices:

- We embrace the concept that patients should receive the most modern and effective advances in care, wrapped in old-fashioned notions about caring. We solve problems and we develop relationships, with equal attention to both.
- We work as a practice team, supporting each other for the benefit of our patients at all levels of care. We will readily terminate any individual who, despite our best efforts at intervention, continues to be poor at working as part of a team.
- We hold the team to performance standards that are high, subject to constant elevation and documented in writing.
- We are a learning company. We believe that each member of the team, no matter how formally or informally educated before arriving here, has more to learn every day. We put large resources of time and money into learning, and we do our best to measure the return on this investment.
- As doctors, managers, and support staff, we tell the truth to each other, even when that truth is difficult or painful, and we stay sufficiently engaged with such discussions to talk out any hurt feelings. We regularly foster a safe space in meetings to air such discussions.
- We seek continuous improvement in the services and products we provide to patients. We also work together to contain costs. It's a really big deal to us when we can discover a protocol change that improves quality without increasing costs or decreases costs without reducing quality.

Owner Support for the Management Team

Administrators and management teams whose decisions are publicly supported by the managing partner and shareholders are generally more willing to make the hard decisions that are periodically necessary by terminating underperforming staff. And the reverse is true.

When the management team believes their recommendation to terminate an employee will be only grudgingly accepted—or worse, actively opposed—even the best managers will withdraw, play it safe, and become tolerant of bad behavior. This creates a vicious cycle, because the best performing staff members will wonder why they are working so hard and following the rules, and their performance will degrade in turn.

Develop organizational standards and communicate these expectations clearly. Spell out expectations in writing so all employees know the practice's expectations and rules, and back these up as often as necessary with verbal reminders (not just occasional admonishments for adverse behavior, but as often as possible, citing favorable, desired behavior when you see it).

Policies and procedures that are consistently enforced have a much stronger impact than those only intermittently enforced.

Consistent Performance Standards for Staff

Most employees want to succeed. They want to perform well and be recognized for it. It's fun to master the job. To do this, expectations and goals must be clear and consistently applied.

For example, if you have an attendance policy with several progressive disciplinary steps leading to termination, you must follow it with no deviation. If you make an exception for the "best tech" because you are sympathetic to her personal issues and she will be hard to replace, you dilute the strength of your own policies and your managers' ability to be effective. Although it can temporarily hurt to terminate an otherwise valuable employee who breaks the rules, you will see the rest of your employees stand up straighter, follow the rules, get you over the short-staffing gap, and, most of all, appreciate that you show no favoritism.

Not Avoiding Confrontation

One thing that makes ophthalmologists generally pleasant to work for is a behavioral style that tends to avoid conflict and confrontation. This can be pleasant in the moment if you work for an ophthalmologist, but it leads to a lot of buried issues in a practice—issues that need to be addressed and improved, but, instead, are avoided. This ophthalmic behavioral style often passes downhill to the management team, so that managers, who need to be confrontational at times, back off.

It's common in our client work to see that the root of poor staff performance is not enforcing reasonable standards because confrontation is culturally uncomfortable in the practice.

Confronting inadequate performance is especially difficult when it involves a long-term, loyal employee who just doesn't have, and will never possess, the skills the practice needs. In cases like this, it is necessary to help reset the owner's ethical compass and resistance to confrontation with a reminder that the owner's highest responsibility is to the patients and to the overall practice, not to the potentially hurt feelings of an individual staff member.

Outside Counsel and Support

Having a labor attorney on speed dial is necessary today, even for the smallest practices. Although, you can get started on your own when a human resources (HR) problem arises by polling your peers or reading HR law articles to understand how others have solved similar problems, how labor laws differ by state, and that missteps are vastly more expensive than the cost of an on-call professional advisor.

You can reduce your HR legal costs with advance preparation. Have notes available while on the call that include:

- The history of the issue
- The relevant practice policies the issue involves
- Steps you have taken (or failed to take) in following applicable policy
- Actions you believe you may want to take
- Any precedent within your practice that could apply

Courage and Planning Pay Off

Firing a staff member can be an emotional step that affects doctors, managers, and staffers alike. Your courage to fire when necessary may be inhibited by your own employment history. Almost everyone working in eye care has been fired or edged out at some time in their career, and it's easy to project your memories onto the current situation. But misapplied empathy only delays the inevitable for the worker and practice.

To alleviate feelings that may be holding you back from the right HR move, be sure you have:

- Followed your written policies to the letter
- Communicated performance standards
- Conducted performance appraisals with concrete feedback, goals, and deadlines
- Provided additional education and training for improvement opportunities
- Documented your efforts and their results
- Consulted with legal counsel and your board where appropriate

If there is still a lapse in performance, you will rest easy knowing that your practice provided every opportunity for the employee to succeed. In retrospect, terminated employees often are happier in new jobs where they have another chance to become successful. Many seasoned supervisors have had the experience of receiving a message from a terminated staffer who months or years later calls to say "thank you" for firing them.

CHAPTER 32

The Importance of Conducting Exit Interviews

Every exit is an entry somewhere else.
—Tom Stoppard

Nobody cares how much you know,
until they know how much you care.
—Theodore Roosevelt

Exit interviewing provides a wealth of information that can improve your practice, keep you in the know, and strengthen critical employee retention efforts. Paradoxically, all too often, the importance of conducting an exit interview in the wake of every employee termination or resignation is overlooked, as if the practice is either afraid to hear what employees may say or, worse, doesn't care.

If performed well, an exit interview sends a very positive message to both exiting and current employees. You show that the practice cares enough to find out why someone wants to leave the organization and in some cases what might have prevented it.

Wohl C, Pinto JB. *UP: Taking Ophthalmic Administrators and Their Management Teams to the Next Level of Skill, Performance, and Career Satisfaction, Second Edition* (pp 169-172).

Exit interviews are especially valuable in settings where turnover rates are higher, let's say above 25% per year in most practices. Conducting an exit interview will help you discern whether there is a deep systemic problem in your practice causing people to leave, or whether resignations are simply beyond your control (spouse relocations and the like).

Performing exit interviews can help you in these ways:

- You will learn staff perceptions about the fairness of workload distribution.
- You will hear feedback on supervisor effectiveness.
- You will perhaps get a more honest sense of how valued and appreciated your employees feel.
- You may learn if written protocols or more communication would have been helpful for employees to feel successful in their roles.
- You will gain a feeling for whether the initial orientation and ongoing training were adequate.

And, they can help you improve how you make hiring decisions in the future. For instance:

____ Does your selection process for hiring include a current position description with the essential skills required?

____ Does your hiring team have a clear understanding of established practice goals to share with the candidates?

____ Is the level of orientation and training commensurate with performance expectations?

____ When you promoted line staff, such as technicians or billers, into management roles did you provide appropriate education and patience as they grew in the new role?

____ What are you learning that will help you modify your hiring practices?

In our experience, most departing employees look forward to sharing their thoughts about the practice or their own jobs during an exit interview. They appreciate that you and the practice care enough to listen to their perspectives and suggestions for improvement that could subsequently help their co-workers.

Exit interviews, performed well, can be empowering to the departing employee. If they hear, truthfully, that their performance was appreciated and their efforts mattered, they leave the practice feeling positive. Consider that what happens during this exit interview will likely be shared with their current peers. We've seen this positive morale booster at the end of their time working with you to be a booster, too, for employees remaining in your employ. And if feelings have not already been hardened, such closing interviews provide an opportunity for you to encourage a departing staffer to send prospective employees your way.

We find that the majority of departing employees are more candid as they prepare to leave because there is less fear of retribution, outside of future reference checks.

There are a variety of methods for conducting such interviews. Our favored method includes using a face-to-face interview, preceded by a short questionnaire.

Here are sample questions you can include in your own written and verbal exit interviews. Of course, the questions will depend of the cause of departure. As with all personnel matters, it is appropriate to run new protocols like this past your labor attorney.

Sample Exit Interview Questions

1. Why are you leaving?
2. If you are going to another job, what does that position offer that your job here does not?
3. Did we meet your expectations as an employer based upon our job posting, interview, and orientation? If not, please explain.
4. Did you suspect or have knowledge of any activities or procedures within the practice that would be in violation of any laws or regulations or that you considered unethical or illegal? If yes, did you report it to someone in authority? To whom? (Note—if this answer is yes, you must follow up more thoroughly on this compliance-related question.)
5. While employed with us did you take any suggestions to your supervisor? If yes, were they followed up to your satisfaction? If not handled satisfactorily, please explain.
6. Rate each of these aspects of your employment here from 1 to 5 (with 1 being terrible and 5 being excellent).
   a. Hourly compensation or salary
   b. Benefits
   c. Supervision
   d. Work conditions
   e. Orientation and training programs
   f. Advancement opportunities
   g. Co-worker friendliness and cooperation
   h. Communication with management
   i. Fair treatment overall by the company

Once you have given your interview subjects an opportunity to collect their thoughts and express them on the questionnaire, you will have a jumping off point for exploration during face-to-face interviews.

Schedule the interview in the middle of the given resignation notice period (eg, 1 week before departure if 2 weeks' notice has been given). This allows for the departing employee to process the acceptance of the change to his or her life while not yet fully disengaged from your practice.

Review the entire form with the departing staffer in detail during the exit interview. At the end of the interview, provide an opportunity to discuss his or her additional thoughts or suggestions.

Who should conduct the interview will differ depending on the size and organizational structure of your practice. It's best for it to not be a direct supervisor, so in the smallest practices we suggest that a doctor or nondirect manager conduct the interview. In larger practices with a deeper mid-level management team, the administrator or HR director is a good choice.

The most fruitful interviews are conducted by an interviewer who:

- Listens more than talks during the interview
- Is not defensive about the employee's perspective or opinion
- Asks for solutions and ideas for any problems mentioned
- Takes good notes that either confirm the departing employee's questionnaire answers or shed new light on why the staffer chose to leave (if it was not a termination)

An important final step is to share the feedback with appropriate management staff and doctors. Take action where indicated by changing policies or learning more about what you heard. If you were asked to keep something confidential, find a way to share the information without breaking the staffer's confidence. For example, if you learned of behaviors you want changed, attempt to place yourself in the position of observing them yourself.

Exit interviews are one of many practice improvement and employee retention tools. They provide a great opportunity to strengthen bonds with both exiting and existing staff, while learning about your practice from an especially candid perspective.

CHAPTER 33

Adding Value to Your Employee Performance Appraisals

When you can't see someone all day long, the only thing you have to evaluate is the work. A lot of the petty evaluation stats just melt away.
—Jason Fried

When we make progress and get better at something, it is inherently motivating. In order for people to make progress, they have to get feedback and information on how they're doing.
—Dan Pink

Those of us who are old enough remember a time when managers and employees could look forward to "evaluation and raise time." Automatic COLAs (cost of living adjustments) were the norm. This was before reimbursements shrank and profit margins tapered. It was a time when salary increases were generous and the performance appraisal process was less precise and less diligent.

Fast forward to our leaner times and the challenges of encouraging employees to be increasingly productive with fewer monetary rewards, having multiple generations of staff working for you who are motivated differently from one another, and needing to find additional ways to retain the best employees.

Wohl C, Pinto JB. *UP: Taking Ophthalmic Administrators and Their Management Teams to the Next Level of Skill, Performance, and Career Satisfaction, Second Edition* (pp 173-176). © 2021 Taylor & Francis Group.

One chief contributor to employee retention is setting clear expectations for job performance up front, and subsequently providing the feedback necessary to recognize achievement or skills gaps.

How can you accomplish this in your practice?

Thought-provoking, meticulously detailed, goal-oriented performance appraisals will add value to your practice. Staff productivity and job satisfaction can be improved when each employee has access to and understands your expectations and sees how one's personal success not only helps the practice flourish, but depends on it.

Perfunctory performance appraisals are boring and unsatisfying for your managers and employees. "Appraisal Lite" can be viewed as a discouraging waste of time, and disappointing for the best staffers who are looking for feedback that helps them grow professionally.

Appraisals that provide little value have become the basis of the recent human resources industry debate on whether performance evaluations provide any value. We hold the opinion that providing clear expectations and prompt feedback for improvements remain valuable to a practice and its employees.

If your performance appraisal process tends to generate a lackluster response, with the exception of, "And now, do I get a raise," your process has room for improvement.

Here are 10 ways that your management team can tune up the evaluation process:

1. Tailor your performance evaluation forms to collaborate with each position description. This helps focus employees on what you are specifically prioritizing within their job duties. By clearly listing what you will prioritize within their overall duties and functions, they are prepared in advance for the skills the practice will be evaluating.
2. Effective evaluations include both objective and subjective components. The objective components must be measurable to clearly communicate the current status and improvement goals. An example would be: "Be able to accurately work up a routine patient in 20 minutes or less." Subjective measures allow you to acknowledge enthusiasm, effort, and insight, and provide discretionary feedback. An example would be: "Patients should report that you answered their questions in a friendly and informative manner."
3. Set three specific goals for each employee, listing the highest of priorities. Include examples of what it will take to achieve each one. For example, rather than stating, "We need you to be a better biller" say "You are currently posting 100 charges daily. Your goal, to be accomplished by September 30th, is to be posting 150 charges daily."
4. Avoid these common weaknesses found in personnel evaluations:
   a. As manager, you score everyone exceptionally high compared to how your management team peers score their staffers. This scoring approach, while it makes staff happy, will limit you in future years. You want to be an accurate scorer, but still leave room for future goals to be acknowledged when reached.
   b. The written details do not include the "what and how" to improve the weaknesses listed. You must be clear about how the weaknesses can be improved. Assume that employees would have fixed their weaknesses on their own if they knew how.

   c. Specific feedback is not provided, particularly if there were previous issues addressed. If you do not know the details, discuss with the employee directly and then complete the form.
   d. Goals or opportunities for improvement are not included. Even the best employees can improve something they already do well. It's okay for goals to include going from good to great.
5. Inexperienced managers and managers who have been poorly supervised during their career can be understandably wary of evaluations. It will help to discuss, in advance, why your practice performs reviews and how valuable you believe they are to improved performance. In your practice, it is not a "gotcha" session, but a formal opportunity for two-way improvement.
6. If everything is a priority, then nothing is prioritized. Establishing communication and goal-setting requirements for your evaluation process will help keep your managers and staff aligned with chief practice goals. This is especially important in fast-growing practices where organizational priorities can get confusing and shift from month to month.
7. Consistent evaluation scoring across the practice can be a challenge. Some managers grade leniently and others grade harder. Management team member philosophies may differ for motivating staff, ranging from giving high praise to leaving scoring room for challenges and growth. Work with your management team to set the parameters you want followed for your practice.
8. Determine your reward system, along with your practice owners, for the accomplishments achieved and to be recognized. Set a budget for salary increases (or bonus ranges) that your management team will work within. Develop standards with your managers for fair distributions. Not all rewards need to be salary-related. Alternate rewards include time off with pay, gift cards, one-time bonuses, and public recognition for excellent achievement.
9. Schedule performance appraisals to be completed by the management team throughout the year. Use the hire date (which becomes the employment anniversary date) as the annual evaluation date for each employee. This spreads the task out over the year for managers. It also takes the focus off "raise time" in the practice. Practices that complete all staff evaluations at the same time annually face the challenge of avoiding salary comparisons among the staff.
10. Conduct at least a mid-year check-up on how each employee is progressing on set goals. Waiting a whole year for feedback can send the wrong messages (eg, these goals aren't that important or your professional growth is not that important to us).

You can apply this focused, goal-setting communication method to other facets of your practice, to providers, and even vendors. Highly successful practices have learned to clearly communicate measurable goals and expectations throughout the organization and provide actionable, encouraging feedback on the progress being made.

• • •

Writing a Flash Appraisal as a Warm-Up for Formal Staff Performance Appraisals

What follows is not a substitute for a formal appraisal, but is a Flash Appraisal we use to help managers and administrators briskly evaluate the people who work under them and think about needed improvements.

Employee	Current Global Score *(0 to 10) **	Potential Maximum Score for This Worker	Potential Activities
Molly (receptionist)	9	10	Continue praise for a job well done, and consider training as the department lead later this year.
Steve (tech)	6	9	Steve has only been on the job 6 months, but it's clear he is going to fit in well here, very bright. Make sure we continue to keep him on a steep learning curve and avoid boredom.
Mary (biller)	5	6	Find Mary's replacement. We need an 8 or higher in this critical function.

*Think of this global score as staffers' overall performance: do they arrive on time, know their job, perform accurately and consistently, work well with others, etc.?

Tip: This same Flash Appraisal is something you can apply to doctors, vendors, and *yourself.*

CHAPTER 34

Setting the Tone of Your Practice Culture

The role of a creative leader is not to have all the ideas; it's to create a culture where everyone can have ideas and feel that they're valued.
—Ken Robinson

Organizational culture refers to the shared values and assumptions of its members. It determines how employees behave in a particular organization. It also affects how the external environment or how people from outside the organization see it. Organizational behavior determines how employees behave ...
—Wikipedia

It's better to hang out with people better than you. Pick out associates whose behavior is better than yours and you'll drift in that direction.
—Warren Buffett

We've all had the experience of walking into a business that makes you feel welcomed, where the employees appear happy and competent and you are served well. Whether it happens in a doctor's office, restaurant, or boutique clothing store, the result is that you will be happy to return, and you tell your friends about your positive experience.

Wohl C, Pinto JB. *UP: Taking Ophthalmic Administrators and Their Management Teams to the Next Level of Skill, Performance, and Career Satisfaction, Second Edition* (pp 177-181).

Positive experiences are greatly impacted by the culture of your practice. And your practice culture affects your employees' behavior and performance. Your patients' experience is an accumulation of the many touch points each meets throughout their visits.

Is the patient experience in your office a result of intention or an accidental accumulation of random, sometimes incongruent, efforts?

A corporation's culture is made up of the collective beliefs and behaviors that drive how a company's employees and management interact and handle outside business transactions. Often, a practice's culture is not expressly or overtly defined, but develops organically over time from the cumulative traits of the people the company hires. However, it's possible to develop an *intentional* culture.

Purposeful, ongoing efforts to set the tone and create a culture you and your patients will enjoy and appreciate not only results in a pleasant environment and great customer service, but it can improve your bottom line. When we see staff and doctors marching in the same direction, we also see efficiency.

When your staff cares and feels cared for, they take the extra steps, go beyond their general position descriptions. They naturally want to ensure smooth processes, cut waste, and offer ideas for improvement. When your culture lacks luster, your staff may show up for work and perform well enough to keep their jobs, but they won't contribute at full potential.

Creating and reinforcing the practice culture you desire starts at the top. The best intended cultural shifts won't endure if your management team is enthusiastic to implement but the owners are lukewarm and not committed. As a leader you must set expectations and clear goals and model the behaviors you want to see in your employees.

Here are 10 steps to help you reinvent your practice culture or take it to the next level:

1. You don't have a coherent culture unless you can describe it in words. Sit down as a group of owners and managers and try to describe your current culture (warts and all) as a collaboration. Writing this description together, with the people present who will be in the position to influence others as you make changes, will increase the odds of success.
2. Document the changes you desire. Written formality is helpful. For example, "Our patients comment that we have lost 'that personal touch' and they now feel like a number. We want our patients to feel recognized and appreciated."
3. Identify the existing barriers that stand between your new goals and the current culture. Perhaps there are unhealthy relationships between certain employees that have been tolerated for years. Or, your onboarding methods are hit and miss, so new hires randomly adopt the culture of their immediate work group rather than the culture you want for the entire practice. Specifically list each issue and brainstorm with your team to develop ways to redo behaviors and adverse values that are holding you back.

4. As you identify issues and barriers, be sure to look deeply and find the root cause of the issues. The problem behind the problem is what likely needs addressing, not the surface issues. For example, if some technicians work nonstop and some are not as busy, perhaps that behavior comes from a former tech manager who encouraged techs to only be of service to the doctor to whom they are assigned each day, rather than be trained and willing to assist with patient flow no matter whose patient it is.
5. Try to hire only new employees who already possess the new values you have set. If your customer services are rated low, help create a new culture of amazing patient satisfaction by hiring staff with great customer service habits from former positions and train them for ophthalmology skills. If you have staff who do not get along with others, hire new employees with an eye for their people skills and check references closely for how they got along with co-workers.
6. If you are in need of a major overhaul of attitudes and behaviors, you may have to replace employees and managers who don't see the benefits of the changes you want to make. New employees can bring fresh ideas to the team and arrive relatively baggage-free. Hanging on to employees unwilling to convert will be discouraging to an enthusiastic and willing staff.
7. Onboard new employees with written formality and an orientation plan specific to each department. A new staffer who spends a day or two with the supervisor and is subsequently provided on-the-job training with an arbitrary employee in the department will be inadequately trained. Make sure you have a written operations manual containing policies and procedures for each job duty, along with a written training schedule that includes timelines for skills developmental. Written protocols can be enforced more fairly and consistently and provide managers a way to hold staff accountable to the standards you and your management team set.
8. For a successful long-term impact, you need to change habits, not just short-term attitudes. Acute team-building efforts and workplace enjoyment strategies belong in this transition but will not be enduring success factors. Enthusiasm has a way of fading, and you don't want your cultural improvements to slip backward. Someone (you as the administrator, or the managing partner, or the department head) has to own the culture of your practice.
9. Engage in quarterly reviews to evaluate the impact of the changes you are making. As a general problem-solving method, you want to:
   a. Collect the data and information (eg, patient satisfaction stats)
   b. Make a data-driven decision (eg, waiting time must be brought down in the morning)
   c. Take action (eg, shift patient slots from morning to afternoon)
   d. Review the action and results. Did it work? And repeat.
10. Be patient. Creating a change in your practice culture does not happen overnight. Your challenge is to eliminate behaviors and attitudes that have been embedded for years. Recognizing which chief issues are holding you back and applying fixes to these priorities is key. Hold the new course you set, make small course corrections along the way, and you'll be on your way to improving not just the performance and sustainability of your practice, but the satisfaction you get from your career.

Ultimately, you and the practice owners have the ability to create an environment where you all love to spend time. Where your patients are well-served. Where your employees are fulfilled and the bottom line shines.

Practice Culture Hallmarks Scorecard

In our experience, the smoothest running and most profitable ophthalmic practices got that way to a large degree because they possess the 10 cultural hallmarks shown. For each of these hallmarks, rate your practice on a 10-point scale, with 0 being "We have none of this attribute" and 10 being "We are the epitome of this attribute." With a possible maximum of 100 points, what is your practice score? Is your score satisfactory or is a lower score holding you back from where you would like to take your practice in the future? What are one or two cultural dimensions you would like to improve?

Hallmark	Score (0 to 10)
1. Our practice is characterized by open, accountable, fearless communication. We don't withhold things from each other. When interpersonal problems or business performance gaps arise, these are quickly addressed and improved.	
2. Our practice is always thinking a few steps ahead and making future plans. Everyone on staff is aware of these plans. Our longer term plans provide a context for making decisions about our daily work priorities.	
3. Teamwork and collaboration is the cultural norm in our practice. Doctors and managers don't solve problems in a vacuum. They have a natural instinct to draw together everyone who is affected by the problem.	
4. Ours is a generous, giving culture at all levels. When a patient is late for an appointment, we extend the benefit of the doubt. Our doctors are generous with patients, spending an extra minute to explain a diagnosis or procedure. We pay our key staff a bit more than they deserve, because this inevitably encourages them to reach for still-higher performance levels.	
5. We universally use positive reinforcement. We see the cup as half full. Patients are told "good job" when they hold still rather than being scolded when they move. Supervisors cite their staff for their good points and their relative improvements.	

(continued)

Hallmark	Score (0 to 10)
6. Each of us as individuals takes responsibility. We don't deflect or blame others or point fingers. This is easy to do because we are not shamed for the mistakes we make, but rather simply encouraged to do better in the future.	
7. Our practice culture is flexible and forgiving. We don't hold grudges. We roll with the punches. We make a fast recovery from setbacks rather than using disappointments as an excuse not to try harder the next time.	
8. Our practice maintains a fast, intense, efficient tempo without appearing hectic, frazzled, or rushed. We don't waste time and are always aware that lost minutes add up, ultimately starving out the financial resources we need to compete effectively, update our facilities, and pay fair wages.	
9. Our practice rolls the dice when it's warranted. We are willing to take reasonable risks. We try new things that may not be sure bets, because we're confident in our ability to recover from misjudgments.	
10. We foster a learning culture here at all levels. We read, attend meetings, hire experts, and visit other practices to learn what works best. We write down protocols so they can be passed uniformly from staffer to staffer. We formally credential and recredential staff.	
Total Score	

CHAPTER 35

Letting Every Worker Help Your Practice Improve

It is not what we get but who we become, what we contribute … that gives meaning to our lives.
—Tony Robbins

Leaders who fail are the ones who do it by themselves. Leaders who succeed are the ones who allow others to help them.
—Simon Sinek

Years ago, Corinne's daughter Rachael had a beloved pet cockatiel. Celery went everywhere with Rachael, tiny claws dug into her shoulder. They happily skipped into the backyard one day, only to come upon the neighborhood cat. Celery leaped for his life, but with clipped wings landed awkwardly on the ground. In a split second, the cat was going in for the kill.

My sweet, kind-hearted 6-year-old instantly and bravely responded by stomping on the cat's tail, scooping up Celery and saving the day. Celery lived many years beyond that incident, safely in the house. And we learned a lesson from Rachael that applies to your practice: *even the least likely person is capable of helpful action.*

Wohl C, Pinto JB. *UP: Taking Ophthalmic Administrators and Their Management Teams to the Next Level of Skill, Performance, and Career Satisfaction, Second Edition* (pp 183-185). © 2021 Taylor & Francis Group.

The reason for sharing this story is to help you recognize that anyone in your practice could step in and save the day, perhaps less dramatically, and help solve a practice problem, even though no one may have anticipated they would or could—or specifically taught them to do so.

It doesn't have to be solely the responsibility of the managing partner or administrator to be the one who sees and adopts new ideas to improve the practice. As an employee of the practice, no matter what your formal title and role, your voice and action can be helpful.

Here are ways to formalize your ideas and share suggestions you have to help strengthen and improve your practice. This list applies to anyone working in your practice.

- **Identify issues along with the potential solutions.** Avoid being the constant complainer who criticizes others' work but offers no alternate solutions. Complainers eventually drown out their own great ideas, which will be dismissed or ignored by others who have learned to tune them out. Instead, bring your concerns to practice leadership along with ways to make improvements. Constructively identify issues and present ideas and research to help the official problem solvers of the practice. For example, if you are frustrated with technicians whose testing results make the doctors uncomfortable, take the time to evaluate the situation. Notice if the inaccuracies occur all the time or only when patient volumes are high. Is it just one tech or many? Whose responsibility is it in your organization to train the technicians? Once you have evaluated and researched the root of the problem, present the facts and your problem-solving ideas to the clinic manager or administrator. You could offer to keep track of the times the problem is at its worse, or to attend the next technician department meeting and provide the education needed to improve their skills. Perhaps skills-building goals for each tech need to be established throughout the practice. Making suggestions—not just lodging your concerns—helps solve problems faster.
- **Be creative.** Most management teams appreciate new ideas, especially when presented with positive intentions. Sometimes it is difficult to see new possibilities, and a fresh approach to a problem will be welcomed. Share creative solutions, especially ones that you've seen work in other settings. For example, do some research with peers across the country. Discover various ways the same problem has been approached in these settings and share these within your practice. Ophthalmic practices are the same the world over. If you have a problem in your practice, a colleague you know has likely tackled it and would be happy to share the solutions he or she found.

- **Make it easier to accept change; call it a trial.** Resistance to change is common, especially if you want to modify a long-standing protocol. Rather than push for a complete overhaul, suggest a multiweek or multimonth trial period and subsequent evaluation to assess the effectiveness of the change. For example, if you do not use a testing schedule template for visual fields or optical coherence tomography scans because you have become accustomed to having the freedom to make it convenient for patients (and yourself) and you can't imagine functioning any other way, but your managers are telling you that total patient waiting time is excessive or that reimbursement may be impacted, you can agree to an adequate trial period and compare the outcomes.
- **Obstacles to excellence.** If you are not in a high position of authority and have identified obstacles that may be diminishing excellence in your practice, determine the best person to approach about it. If it's a clinic flow problem, start with the clinic manager. If it is a broader issue, for example, total transit time for your patients on a daily basis, gather the details and discuss it with your administrator or managing partner. If you detect an overall dissatisfaction among your peers about the lack of educational opportunities within the practice, offer to head a new task force that will develop ideas to solve this problem. It is generally encouraged in well-run practices to follow the chain of command to problem solve. But the best practices also encourage continued, up-the-ladder follow-up if the problem remains unsolved.
- **A safe environment.** To feel comfortable offering your opinion or new ideas, the environment needs to feel safe. In practices where there is a feeling that "no one makes suggestions here" a likely contributing factor is a history of leadership not respecting new ideas or giving them lip service but not implementing them. Micromanaged and overcontrolled environments can lead to employees feeling disheartened about the prospect of their ideas ever being heard or seriously considered. If you are in a leadership position and your practice feels closed or hostile to new ideas, ask if there is an opportunity to foster more safety and openness.
- **Be brave enough to learn what your staff really thinks**. One of the best ways to determine how employees feel is to perform an anonymous employee opinion survey. Such surveys help assess employee perceptions and provide you with an objective basis for prioritizing and addressing their concerns. And don't just let such surveys languish after they are completed. Share the results with all staff. Act vigorously to install the best ideas.

CHAPTER 36

The Business Benefits of Workplace Enjoyment

I am going to keep having fun every day I have left, because there is no other way of life. You just have to decide whether you are a Tigger or an Eeyore.
—Randy Pausch

When you have confidence, you can have a lot of fun. And when you have fun, you can do amazing things.
—Joe Namath

If you obey all the rules you miss all the fun.
—Katharine Hepburn

We worked with a practice manager on the East Coast recently who shared in confidence, "I don't know how to have fun." (He didn't even say it with a smile.) And thus started an interesting, 3-day dialog on the economics of workplace fun.

The greatest operating cost in your practice, irrespective of scale, is staff—both lay staff and any associate care providers you employ. In the typical setting, 30% or more of every dollar you collect goes to employed staff.

Curating a practice team and managing providers and support staff well involves numerous aspects:

Wohl C, Pinto JB. *UP: Taking Ophthalmic Administrators and Their Management Teams to the Next Level of Skill, Performance, and Career Satisfaction, Second Edition* (pp 187-190).

- Correct hiring choices
- Written performance standards
- Great, never-ending training
- Fair, frequent performance feedback
- Appropriate discipline and redirection
- Not delaying termination decisions

Which brings us back to those very un-businesslike concepts—"fun," "enjoyment," "happiness"—words that are not often on a punch list of staff management pearls. They should be. The absence of workplace enjoyment is the key driver for staff dissatisfaction and excessive turnover. And excessive turnover has some very high, hard costs in the ophthalmic United States. In the typical ophthalmic practice today, the average turnover rate (the percent of staff who leave each year for one reason or another) is about 25%. In practices that make an active effort to reduce this figure, 15% is the norm. In lower morale settings, the annual turnover rate can be 35% or higher.

What does this cost in dollars? According to labor economists, the cost to a company of losing one staff member is about 50% of that person's annual wage. This rule-of-thumb estimate includes the cost to recruit, hire, and train a replacement worker, plus the lost productivity and extra burdens put on the staff left behind.

Here's an example. Imagine a three-surgeon practice with 24 lay staff. The normal turnover rate would be 25%, or about six people departing per year. If this same practice had disgruntled, unhappy employees, and the turnover rate was 38%, or nine departing staff instead of six, the cost associated with the excess staff departures would be: three excess staff, times their $45,000 average wage, times a 50%-of-wage cost, equals $67,500. In a practice this size, three excess staff leaving in a year could represent a 5% or greater reduction in profitability.

• • •

Great staff management certainly takes wise hires and great supervision. But it also takes fun.

The fun factor in a practice comes from the top. When the administrator and surgeons are playful by nature, it rolls downhill to the rest of the staff. Unfortunately, doctors and administrators can be notoriously uncheerful. They are serious people doing serious work. Being serious is what got them elevated to this level of authority. If this is you, here's a helpful combo menu of fun, disarming, and nearly cost-free actions you can take to boost workplace enjoyment for staff and doctors alike.

- Budget and delegate for fun. Choose two nonsupervisory staff for the year to collaborate on fun activities and give them a budget.
- Memorize one joke per week. Learn how to tell it well ... or not. You can tell it poorly. In fact, the more uptight and stuffy you are seen to be by your staff, the more hilarious and appreciated your efforts will be.
- Learn a magic trick or two. Dr. Spencer Thornton, one of the most smiling ophthalmologists we know, has spread joy to staff and patients alike with magic. Even a bungled trick will raise the fun factor.

- Don't overlook any opportunity to dress up (and be chuckled at). Wear costumes or fun accessories for Halloween, Thanksgiving, Valentine's Day, and other holidays.
- Dress up the office, too. You should have a plastic tub in storage for each of the holidays, along with one or two holidays that you make up. (How about celebrating "Half-Way Day" when half of the year is done? Or "Half-Million Day" when you've served your 500,000th patient?)
- Create traditions and celebrate them. (Honoring the most cheerful and upbeat person in the office in the last month with a small smiley button to wear.)
- This one is easy and highly effective: Feed people free food. You should bring in lunch, snacks, dessert, pastries, or the like at least once per week on a random schedule.
- Increase workplace enjoyment by loosening up your instructions. Nobody likes to be told precisely, in exquisite detail, *how* to do their job. People like to know the outcomes you expect of them and have a chance to innovate their own way to the desired outcome.
- As the administrator or lead physician in your practice, be extremely sensitive to interpersonal conflicts. Don't allow them to simmer with hopes that the conflicts will fade away. These will always arise in a workplace, but they should cool down briskly. Your job as a leader is to reduce the level of conflict wherever it arises. Conflict kills work enjoyment.
- Without going over the line, without trying to be a buddy, be accessible to staff. Providers and administrators should treat line staff not like peers (you're not), but like respected colleagues with important roles to play in a common mission. Don't treat staff like minions beneath you.
- Preserve and strictly enforce all the important rules (eg, patient safety, clocking in, name tags) while relaxing others (eg, a relaxed dress code on Fridays).
- Keep a sharing library of audiobooks for staff (without podcast access) who have long commutes to borrow.
- Launch a company fitness club, walking group, or bowling or softball team.
- Allow staff to personalize their workspace with photos, vacation memorabilia, etc.
- Decorate the break room whimsically. Hire a singing telegram for hallmark employment anniversaries. Do not forget birthdays! Cakes, a card, an internal newsletter announcement are all avenues to help celebrate.
- Don't let doctors intervene with staff about performance errors; make sure these all get filtered through the appropriate supervisor.
- The administrator and managing partner should take at least one complete walking tour of the office daily, each visiting casually with staff in all areas and praising them about specific aspects of their performance. If necessary, arrive early or stay late to accomplish this.
- Check local wages to ensure pay equity in all areas of the practice.
- When you have especially tough or late days, consider "battle pay," meritorious service awards, compensatory time off, and the like.

- Find ways to increase scheduling flexibility for staff. Start by asking staff what changes in scheduling would make their lives easier while still delivering great patient care and customer service.
- The administrator should take two different staffers to lunch each week to listen and learn, both up and down the chain of command.
- Doctors: Share your future dreams for the practice. Most staff see their work as a career and want to know where you are taking them as their leader.
- Make sure any final job candidates (including doctors) are interviewed briefly by every staff member (or by as many as practical in large practices).
- And finally, Google "workplace fun" for about 87 million other ideas of how to boost staff enjoyment of their jobs.

CHAPTER 37

Human Resources Issues

What Should I Do When ...?

Holding on to anger is like grasping a hot coal with the intention of throwing it at someone else—you are the one who gets burned.
—Buddha

Speed is everything. It is the indispensable ingredient of competitiveness.
—Jack Welch

HR Challenge and Tip #1: Address HR Issues Promptly and With the Management Infrastructure Needed to Do So

Quickly address human resources (HR) conflicts. Direct, appropriate confrontation can be awkward, uncomfortable, even painful. But ultimately you find that resolving conflict promptly is a relief for all employees (directly or indirectly impacted) and creates a healthier, more productive environment.

Delayed decisions and actions impact not only the current bottom line but future financial opportunity as well. It is possible to be a strong leader, financially

Wohl C, Pinto JB. *UP: Taking Ophthalmic Administrators and Their Management Teams to the Next Level of Skill, Performance, and Career Satisfaction, Second Edition* (pp 191-194).

responsible, and treat colleagues and employees well. Below are a few ways to be sure you have an organizational structure in place to address HR issues.

- The administrator or office manager needs the credentials, education, and/or appropriate experience for the job you expect of them. Sometimes the practice's success pace outgrows the current talent. Recognize and manage the level of management talent you need. For example, managing six staff members is very different than managing 20 or more.
- If you are a doctor leading the practice yourself and have little experience managing HR issues, use outside advisors like your labor attorney or practice consultant. They've heard it all before and can guide you at a small cost, compared to expensive rookie errors we all make when inexperienced at a task. Another option is an arrangement with a noncompetitive practice to share an administrator if you both don't need one full time. (This solution could assist you with more areas than just HR.)
- Avoid emotion. Easier said than done. Handling HR issues emotionally can lead you down the wrong path. These are business decisions and although you can approach them with professionalism, caring, and kindness, leading the problem-solving task with emotion can get you in trouble.
- Creating committees or teams to address practice-wide issues helps with buy-in for policy changes. Including the right people in the decision-making process can ensure that all the information needed will be collected. As important, it provides the needed support for an effective change, especially one that is controversial. Have you noticed that when solutions are not always handed down from above, but created during a process that includes the employees or doctors involved in implementation, fresh ideas, solutions, and even alternate perspectives arise?
- Expect pushback from staff after implementing a tough decision made to benefit the practice more directly than individual employees. Hold strong and don't backtrack, unless after reevaluation you choose to make adjustments. Support each other's management decisions and be viewed as a collaborative team that means business. Make decisions based on the best direction for the practice, not necessarily individuals. In the end, the practice will be stronger, benefiting all.

HR Challenge and Tip #2: Tackling Conflict

The obvious reason many doctors and managers dread HR issues is because they can be very tricky to solve. There always seem to be unique circumstances. Possible solutions are often restricted and/or guided by law, sometimes making it feel like possible solutions go against common sense. Personal emotions can be barriers toward the best business decision, although they can also be a compass for you.

Newer managers are often technically accomplished, but most challenged by HR issues. So are doctors without management training, because what seems logical or clear to a non-HR experienced person is often just part of the answer, not covering the myriad possible side effect outcomes. With experience and applied consistency, HR issues can be tackled with confidence and success. You may even end up enjoying these challenges! The following are two common HR issues along with suggested approaches:

1. **We have two managers who always seem to disagree with each other. It creates conflict and discomfort in our practice environment.**
    - Assess the situation with fresh objectivity. Meet with each one individually, asking each the same questions. Why do you often disagree with Manager Other? Is there a professional or personal component to the issue? Is it competition, lack of respect, or understanding for each other's position, long-timer vs new-timer issues? What do you think can be done to resolve this conflict?
    - How are their actions impacting employees and, ultimately, patient care?
    - Once you determine the underlying issues, create a solution path and develop a written plan. Be very specific with the expectations you give each manager.
    - Meet with both at the same time. Clearly communicate your expectations and how each will be held accountable. For example, they must work in conjunction with each other in supporting roles. You expect them to keep conflicts to themselves and not share with staff. If conflicts crop up, they will handle them together, professionally, for the benefit of the practice, fellow employees and patients. You expect them to work through problems together first, only involving you after they've tried.
    - They will bring any unresolved matters to the administrator or managing partner in a timely manner, not allowing an issue to fester beyond repair.
    - Success or failure, after the expectations are clarified, will be reflected in their annual performance appraisals. Changes in behavior and insight that benefit the practice will be rewarded.
2. **A manager often does not complete work in a timely fashion.**
    - Assess the situation objectively. Is this a new phenomenon or has it always been this way? Can you pinpoint when it changed? Was there a corresponding organizational shift (eg, staffing changes, new responsibilities, new doctor or service line added)?
    - Ask yourself if you give clear direction on due dates and project expectations. If not, your manager may not even be aware of missing the mark you have in mind.
    - Address your concern directly with the manager. Provide specific examples of how established deadlines are not being met and ask his or her perspective on what the barriers have been.
    - Listen closely to the answers. You may learn something about the practice that you've not appreciated before. It's common for us to think we know all the answers. But practice management is complicated and small, undetected details (eg, barriers) can make a difference in the way employees can perform (or think they are allowed perform).
    - Ask yourself if your expectations are realistic. Are there too many projects on the manager's plate? It's better to set three to five goals, have them met, and set three to five more, as opposed to having 25 projects listed on which a manager flounders while working on them all at once.

- Are task and project deadlines written and communicated? Use meeting minutes or project planning tools for clarification.
- If it ultimately is an individual performance issue, proceed the commonly recommended way for addressing employee performance issues. Set clear, written expectations. Agree on goals and timelines together. Follow up promptly if the deadline is not met and find out why. Be open to adjusting the timeline when good reasons to do so are present. Document the success or failure of meeting the deadline for the manager. Be prepared to replace the manager, if needed. And if you replace the manager, you will know that you provided a fair opportunity to succeed.

Section VI

Meaningful Measurements

Benchmarking Key Performance Indicators

CHAPTER 38

Math

Your Second Language as Administrator

The essence of mathematics is not to make simple things complicated, but to make complicated things simple.
—Stanley Gudder

The only way to learn mathematics is to do mathematics.
—Paul Halmos

Psychologist Sian Beilock at the University of Chicago has explained why math is so uncomfortable for some people. Apparently the mental anguish math-adverse people feel is sourced to the same ancient, evolutionarily, primitive area of our brains—the dorsal posterior insula that is activated when we experience bodily, physical pain.

In math-phobes, research has shown that just the mere *thought* of having to do math is enough to light up this region of the brain on scans. This study has important consequences in the sphere of practice administration, because the clearest dividing line between good and great administrators is their comfort with math.

Wohl C, Pinto JB. *UP: Taking Ophthalmic Administrators and Their Management Teams to the Next Level of Skill, Performance, and Career Satisfaction, Second Edition* (pp 197-199).

We know many otherwise very bright office managers who have been stuck for years at a level barely above clerk because of weak math skills. For them, math is a kind of impenetrable second language they can't seem to learn. Just the act of trying to puzzle out a business math problem hurts.

If you want to be a great ophthalmic business leader, and make the leap from clerk or manager to administrator, it is essential that you learn to think like the doctors who employ you, which is to engage bravely with the world of objective facts and data.

Medicine, after all—particularly the ophthalmic kind—is largely about numbers:

- A refraction generates a numeric prescription.
- An intraocular pressure check yields two numbers, one for each eye.
- Even cataracts are graded on a numeric scale.

Much has changed since John started consulting in ophthalmology more than 40 years ago. Back then "Patient doing fine" was a perfectly acceptable and complete chart note. Back then, an equally subjective business performance report was also acceptable: "Billing is all caught up."

Everyone is at least a little anxious about math, just like we are all a little anxious about flying or public speaking, no matter how much of it we do. That's normal. But practice administrators who are truly math-phobic are as held back in their careers as administrators who can't stand up in front of the staff to give a training session or fly to a national symposium.

Experts say that severe phobia is a learned anxiety. No one is born afraid of flying or speaking or doing math. Your dislike for math is probably rooted in a belittling teacher or parent. Nearly all of us over a certain age have had the experience of being called up to the blackboard to solve a math problem with our classmates looking on. (For some of you, just reading this last sentence may still give you the chills!)

And if you're a woman, this may have been reinforced by the slow-dying social myth that "girls are innately not very good at math." Unlearning any debilitating anxiety is not a matter of suppressing or denying the phobia. It's more constructive to own your anxiety, to not be self-critical, and to take steps to overcome it.

Here are three approaches to overcoming math anxiety.

First, realize that most business math is pretty simple. Sure, calculus and higher-order statistics are used in large corporate settings, but the basic arithmetic you studied in grammar school is all you need to understand and solve most practice-based business problems.

There are only two species of numbers for you to master, both pretty easy. One set of numbers is primary: the number of patient visits seen in the clinic, for example, or the month-by-month collections. The other set of numbers are derivatives. Most practice benchmarks fall into this category. Examples include:

- The average ticket (monthly collections divided by monthly patient visits)
- Surgical density (monthly visits divided by monthly surgical cases)
- Tech efficiency (monthly tech payroll hours divided by monthly visits)

As you can see, there's nothing more complex here mathematically than simple long-hand division. You could have done these kinds of math problems when you were about 10 years old.

The biggest boost to understanding business math may not come from deciphering rows of abstract figures, but from turning numbers into pictures. Take a glance at these two formats for looking at practice profits. Which is more readily understandable?

	Annual Profit
2011	250,000
2012	243,000
2013	315,000
2014	375,000
2015	485,000
2016	695,000
2017	625,000
2018	600,000

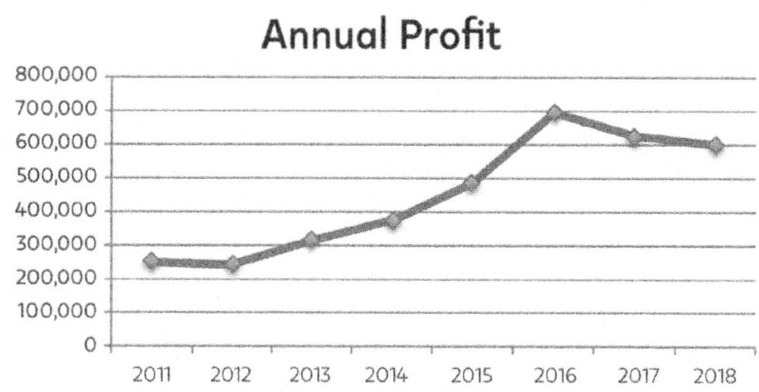

Second, talk to your managing partner or solo practice owner. Odds are he or she is pretty good at math or else would not have made it through training. Most of the eye surgeons we know enjoy teaching when approached the right way, and there's a hidden bonus: the kind of business math you need to master as an administrator may not be all that familiar to your doctor, either. Make better business numeracy a challenge you work on together.

Last, harness your practice's accounting and consulting resources. Ask them to teach you how to read the monthly financial statements and how to calculate the most relevant benchmarks each quarter. Realize that just as your doctors turn to outside specialists at the local university and their peers to help them solve tough clinical cases, it's perfectly okay for you to turn to outside advisors when you're stumped with an unaccustomed round of business analysis.

As Bleilock and her colleagues discovered, "It's not that math itself hurts. Rather, merely the anticipation of math is painful." So, the conclusion is clear if you are math-phobic: face your fear of math and do it anyway. Just starting your computations will help the pain subside.

CHAPTER 39

Critical Numbers for Data-Driven Decision Making

The key is not to prioritize what's on your schedule, but to schedule your priorities.
—Stephen Covey

Statistics are no substitute for judgment.
—Henry Clay

Imagine we erased from ophthalmology textbooks and training programs just a few critical numbers. Let's say, refractive error, intraocular pressure, and cup-to-disc ratio. Poof. Gone.

This isn't much information compared to the thousands of factoids your doctors had to master to become a physician, right? Way less than 1% of what they had to learn. And yet, the absence of just these three metrics would set them back 99%, to the ranks of a 19th century ophthalmologist.

Those three numbers are so central to the profession that we could stop any doctor in your practice on any clinic day, and they'd be able to rattle off these three numbers on the last patient seen.

Wohl C, Pinto JB. *UP: Taking Ophthalmic Administrators and Their Management Teams to the Next Level of Skill, Performance, and Career Satisfaction, Second Edition* (pp 201-212).

The same is true in the business of ophthalmology, where there is just one "patient," the practice itself, and you are the practice's "doctor." Competent administrators and department managers commit to memory the norms for numerous key performance indicators and know by rote what the values are for their practice or department at any one time.

Here are several metrics as critical to evaluating the economic health of your practice as intraocular pressure is to evaluating a patient's eye health. As a practice administrator or owner, how many of these do you know off the top of your head without looking at reports?

- **Practice growth rate.** Although the US population is growing at only about 1% per year, the demand for ophthalmic services is growing at about 4% per year. This is because the population of older adults is growing at three times the pace of the overall population, and older adults (happily for us in eye care) need a lot more of our services compared to younger patients. Growth rate, in revenue terms, is simple to calculate. A practice collecting $1 million per year that grows by $50,000 in 12 months is growing at a 5% pace. A practice growing more than 4% per year is likely gaining market share. Not only should you know your current growth rate, but you should have an agreed-upon growth rate target in the board room.
- **Patient visits per doctor per month.** This is simply the total average monthly visits (including postoperative patients) for each provider in your practice. Typical figures are 550 or more in a hardworking general ophthalmologist's office, 450 or more in most subspecialty settings. This benchmark is vital because in a fixed-cost business like ophthalmology, profit enhancement is more often a matter of revenue enhancement than cost containment. In a solo practice, seeing just three extra patients per clinic day can boost annual collections by $100,000 or more. You would have to terminate more than two lay staff to achieve the same profit result, which would then likely harm the practice due to understaffing.
- **Average collections per patient visit.** This is also called the *average ticket*, which varies widely from setting to setting, and across the subspecialties. Simply divide total annual collections (net of drug collections if you have a retinal practice or have a comprehensive generalist performing retinal injections) by annual patient visits (including postoperative visits). This measurement can be taken for the overall practice or for each individual provider. In a general, cataract practice, the typical range is $150 to $225 or slightly more. There are several factors influencing this metric. The most important are the underlying nature of the practice and the clinical and surgical assertiveness of the providers. Practices serving an older/sicker patient population will have a higher average ticket. Practices with a high co-management component that primarily perform surgery will have a higher average ticket. Practices with a high primary care component will have a lower average ticket unless optical and contact lens sales are emphasized.

- **Surgical density.** Various advisors measure this in different ways, but the convention we use is to divide average monthly patient visits (including postoperative visits) by average monthly surgical cases. In the typical, middle-of-the-road anterior segment practice, we would find a practice with 550 visits and ±25 cataracts a month, well within the typical surgical density range of 10 to 30 visits per case. A purely co-managing practice may transit just five visits per surgery. A young surgeon just getting started may only have a mild surgical density of 50 visits per case and be perfectly normal.
- **Profit margin.** While there are several useful conventions for measuring profitability, the most common for a medical practice is to divide total MD or DO annual profits (including wages, taxes, benefits, dividends, officer entitlements, and the like) by total practice collections (again, net of drug collections). The typical range today in a general practice is 30% to 45%. A generation ago, this was 35% to 50% or higher, so margins are falling. Aside from the obvious benefit to practice owners, a higher profit margin practice is a safer practice, with better odds of survival in the event of deeper fee cuts, provider loss, or competitor encroachment.
- **Staffing costs as a percent of cash flow.** The highest cost center in virtually every practice is lay staffing. Add up all employment costs (wages, taxes, benefits) and divide by net practice collections. A $1 million practice in net collections, spending $300,000 per year on staff, would have a 30% staffing cost. Norms are 28% to 32% in general practices, slightly less in retinal practices, and somewhat more in urban practices where wages are generally higher. If you are at 35% or higher, the most likely reason is overstaffing or excessive wages. Just like a patient's medical condition, you will have to judge if you should treat the problem or live with it.
- **Established patient growth rate.** This is one of the most overlooked opportunities discovered in the typical new client practice. In a general ophthalmology practice, the number of established patients (total patients minus new patients) should be growing by about 5% per year. A practice with established patient growth rates below 5% (or worse, a negative growth rate) commonly has one of two chief problems: either a flawed recall system or customer service gaps.

If some of these key performance indicators stumped you, it's time to make up some flash cards and take yourself back to school. Once you master these calculations, go for extra credit with the following basic and advanced benchmarking examples and exercises.

Basic Benchmarking Examples and Exercises: Productivity and Efficiency Benchmark Examples

Basic Example #1: Doctors

Count the number of patient visits (including postoperative visits) your entire practice sees in a typical month. Then divide this patient count by the number of doctor equivalents (DEs). A DE is one physician working full time or two optometrists working full time.

Example:

- Two surgeons and 1 optometrist, all working full time, are 2.5 DEs
- These doctors see 1350 patients per month
- 1350 visits divided by 2.5 DEs equals 540 visits per DE per month

What's your number? ______________

Basic Example #2: Exam Rooms

Count the number of fully equipped and active exam rooms in your practice. Multiply this number by 173 (the number of hours of operation in the typical practice). Divide the resulting figure into the number of total patients (including postoperative) seen in a month.

Example:

- The previous 1350-patient-per-month practice has 8 active exam rooms
- 1350 visits divided by 1384 room-hours (8 rooms × 173 hours) equals 1.0 patient visit per room hour

What's your number? ______________

Basic Example #3: Technicians

Count the number of technician full-time equivalents (FTEs) in your practice. (An FTE is one staffer working 40 hours per week. Someone working 20 hours per week would be 0.5 FTE.) Count as techs anyone who is rooming and working up patients, assisting chair side, or performing special testing. Multiply the resulting FTE count by 173 (the number of paid payroll hours in the typical month) and divide the resulting number by the number of patient visits per month.

Example:

- The 1350-patient-per month practice has 6.5 tech FTEs
- 1125 tech hours (6.5 FTEs × 173 hours) divided by 1350 visits equals 0.8 tech payroll hour per patient visit

What's your number? ______________

Basic Example #4: Patient Accounts Staff

Count the number of billing staff FTEs in your practice. Count as billing anyone who is securing authorization, posting charges, submitting claims, posting payments, chasing denials, submitting secondary claims, handling collections, and all the other myriad details that go with this tangled labyrinth in your practice. Multiply the resulting FTE count by 173 and divide the resulting figure by the number of total monthly transactions (for ease, typically the patient visits plus the surgical cases).

Example:

- The 1350-visit (and let's say 70 cataract) practice has 2.5 billing staff FTEs
- 433 billing staff hours (2.5 FTEs × 173 hours) divided by 1420 transactions (1350 visits plus 70 surgeries) equals 0.3 billing staff payroll hour per transaction

What's your number? ______________

Basic Exercise #5: Reception/Clerical Staff

Count the number of clerical staff FTEs in your practice. Include anyone who is checking patients in or out, handling the phone lines, or keeping the medical records tidy. Exclude personal secretaries and transcriptionists. Multiply the resulting FTE count by 173 and divide the resulting number by the number of total monthly patient visits.

Example:

- The 1350-visit practice above has 3.0 reception staff FTEs
- 519 billing reception hours (3.0 FTEs × 173 hours) divided by 1350 visits equals 0.4 reception/clerical staff payroll hour per transaction

What's your number? ______________

Your results for an efficient, productive general ophthalmologist should be roughly in line with the previous sample practice with:

- 500 or more patient visits per DE per month
- Between 0.7 and 1.1 patient visits per exam room per hour
- Between 0.8 and 1.0 tech payroll hours per patient visit
- Plus or minus 0.3 billing staff payroll hours per transaction
- About 0.5 receptionist payroll hours per patient visit

Advanced Benchmarking Exercises

The goal is to move beyond the common approach of collecting data, reporting benchmarks, and approaching and analyzing them one at a time. Let's take a look at a deeper set of benchmarks, with a more sophisticated interpretation that ultimately enhances their value.

Advanced Exercise #1: How Is Our Billing Department Performing?

The situation:

- 12-surgeon comprehensive practice
- Four full-time office locations
- Billing handled in main office
- Batch posting in billing department
- Electronic health records, but three senior doctors don't use scribes and don't complete charting same day
- Compliance plan and officer, but no external auditing for past 5 years
- Billing department manager is also responsible for overseeing three satellite offices
- Billing department manager reports to administrator (former hospital executive) who has strong finance background but poor understanding of revenue cycle management (RCM)
- No collection agency; late accounts are written off aggressively to help department manager receive her bonus

The data:

- Fast-growing practice (@16% >3 × demand growth)
- Service-to-charge posting takes up to 4 days (tardy doctors and superbills find their way to main office slowly)
- 72,000 visits per year (and growing!)
- 8000 major surgical cases per year
- 9.7 department FTEs
- Department staff turnover rate is 35%
- Open ticket report is generated periodically but not interpreted
- Aging report shows open accounts over 90 days at 8%
- Net collection ratio is 85%

Interpretation:

- With 80,000 transactions per year and 9.7 FTEs in the billing department, we have 0.25 billing staff payroll hours per transaction; norms would be ±0.3, so on paper the department is about 17% understaffed.
- The billing department manager should be 100% dedicated to RCM; satellite office operations oversight is a distraction.

- Understaffing in the department is made worse by four factors:
  1. Less than fully dedicated department head
  2. Fast growth of the practice
  3. High turnover of the department staff (it can take years to become competent in this practice area; departing staff walk away with legacy skills that are hard to immediately replace)
  4. Doctor tardiness with charting
- Four-day delay from date of service to date of posting is two to four times longer than typical.
- In a practice with paperwork-tardy doctors, the open ticket report can help pinpoint the laggards.
- Many practices with dispersed operations (and even those with just one office) have shifted to charge posting at checkout to accelerate cash flow.
- While the 8% >90-day open accounts statistic is favorable, it comes at the cost of rushed write-offs.
- The 85% net collection ratio should be 95% or higher.

The plan:

- Elevate department staffing from 9.7 to 11.5 FTEs, which will normalize labor productivity to 0.3 hours per transaction.
- In adding staff, make sure that all department workers have a quiet space to do their work (not in a practice thoroughfare).
- Shift billing manager's satellite operations management duties to designated on-site managers; focus 100% on billing department.
- Provide RCM training for the administrator. In a practice this size, the administrator needs to know how to post a charge, submit a claim, and run and interpret reports. This becomes somewhat less critical as the practice grows and billing department has a deeper bench.
- Consider shift from batch posting of charges to posting at check-up (adding training and hours in reception as needed).
- Generate open ticket report weekly and establish board-level policy that providers must close out their charts on the same day, except for exceptional circumstances.
- Write protocols obliging billing staff to optimize fee recovery. Don't write off fees that are recoverable.
- Monitor net collection ratio; live with the somewhat elevated open accounts over 90-day statistic.
- Engage a specialist for a baseline charting and coding audit and department review; repeat every 1 to 3 years depending on findings.

Advanced Exercise #2: Is It Time to Add Another Provider? Which Kind?

The situation:

- 45-year-old solo ophthalmologist
- 5-year lease can't be broken
- Making 30% margin on $756,000 in annual collections, $227,000 personal income
- MD would like a pay raise

The data:

- Working 4.5 days per week (4.0 in clinic)
- Five exam rooms
- 520 visits per month
- Growing 10% annually
- Five-week wait for the next routine appointment
- Fifteen cataracts per month
- Average preoperative/pre–brightness acuity test best corrected visual acuity (BCVA)=20/67
- $63,000 in monthly collections

Interpretation:

- At 520 visits, MD is at about 95% of a soloist's capacity.
- With 5 lanes, at 60% of office capacity; growing 10% annually, will need more space in about 5 years.
- 520 visits/15 cases=35 visits/case=low surgical density (with average BCVA of 20/67=30% more conservative than typical cataract surgeon).
- $63,000/520 visits=very low $121 average ticket (due to low surgical density and low testing rates).
- If a second MD added, not enough income to support two doctors for many years … steep pay cut.
- If the chief complaint is insufficient MD income, adding another provider will make the problem worse.
- The top priority is to increase collections per visit and boost incremental volumes to get this MD up to full capacity, not adding another doctor.

The plan:

- Increase template to allow 30 more visits per month (about $50,000 annual pay raise).
- Increase surgical density of the practice; 550 visits should yield 22 cases or more per month (find a surgeon mentor to ramp up assertiveness).
- Examine Current Procedural Terminology report for testing gaps.
- Examine RCM for collection gaps.

- With continued growth, add a part-time OD when MD is at full capacity in about 12 months.
- Make a decision about adding facilities in 4 years.

Advanced Exercise #3: Should We Expand Our Current Facilities or Open a Satellite?

The situation:

- Four MD, two OD group practice
- One suburban location at full facility capacity
- Half of the board wants to stay in one location and expand
- Half of the board wants to relieve the facility pressure by opening a rural satellite 15 miles away

The data:

- Practice currently sees 2125 visits per month with 5 DEs. 425/DE-mo., 77% of capacity (DE = 1 MD or 2 ODs).
- Current location is saturated with only 15,000 people per ophthalmologist (norms ≥ 20,000).
- Current location has 14% older adults (US norms).
- Potential rural market has 35,000 people per MD and 18% older adults (about 70% underserved).
- One of the practice ODs lives in the rural market.

Interpretation:

- Practice is overdoctored in the current office.
- Current patient base could be handled by 4 DEs.
- Current providers could readily see another 625 patients per month (but not in the current office facilities without evening/weekend hours).
- Every office location should have a "homeroom" doctor, and the local OD would be a perfect fit for this role (it reduces the OD's commute).

The plan:

- It is almost certainly better to open the satellite but prepare a pro forma to confirm economics.
- Write a 10-year plan spelling out how this satellite fits into the big picture.
- Lease a "beachhead" office for now (expand later).
- Name a lay site manager to work alongside the local OD (who will be homeroom doctor).
- Rotate suburban MDs through the rural office.
- Remember: Two locations will quadruple complexity. Make sure the managers are ready.

Advanced Exercise #4: What Should We Do About the Drop in Our Patient Visits?

The situation:

- $7.5 million comprehensive, dispensing practice; a local leader in a growing retirement community.
- Five owners.
- 2% revenue growth in prior year.
- Expenses rose 3%; profits flat.
- Some of the owners want to launch a new $350,000 direct to consumer campaign proposed by a local ad agency to increase patient visits.

The data:

- Established patients down 4% in the last year
- Average collections per visit: $205
- Surgical cases increased by 5%
- 35% clerical staff turnover last 12 months
- 10% of surgical cases are referred by external ODs
- No-show rate is 8%
- 7.0 reception/phone/records staff FTEs
- Appointment book kept out 6 months
- Practice spends 2% of cash flow on marketing, mainly on newspaper ads and billboards

Interpretation:

- With $7.5 million in collections and an average ticket of $205, this practice sees 36,585 visits per year, so we need 8.8 reception/phone/medical records staff (0.5 hours/visit).
- We only have 7.0 staff (0.40 hours/visit) in a department with high turnover, so skill and productivity are likely at half of norms.
- This in turn likely drives recall effectiveness down, exacerbated by only booking out 6 months and recalling all other patients.
- Established patient volumes should grow 5% per year, not shrink 4% as happened last year.
- The 9% established patient spread times about 31,000 established patients in the baseline year, means we dropped about $570,000 in revenue last year because of poor continuity of care, a nearly 8% revenue gain.
- Practice revenue grew only 2% last year, when market demand probably grew 5%, the practice lost market share.
- But, spending more on external marketing is not the answer.
- This case points out the most common error in responding to a decrease in patient visits: not realizing that continuity of care and recall are marketing job #1.

The plan:

- Recall audit to identify gaps (MDs not nominating a firm return-to-clinic order, front desk defaulting to recall).
- Staff up reception and firm up protocols.
- Book templates out a perpetual 12 months or more and book all such exams (sharply limit recall notices).
- Call lost patients from prior loose recall years.
- Reexamine current marketing and redeploy existing budget, as needed, until continuity of care (internal marketing) is improved and stabilized.

Advanced Exercise #5: How to Calculate the Critical Components in a Practice

The situation and data:

The staff and doctors of Wobegone Eye Center (WEC) decide to go on a holiday weekend retreat, leaving the practice in the hands of the administrator's new executive assistant and the just-hired MD associate. Unfortunately, as a cost-saving measure, the administrator of WEC chartered a plane with faulty mechanics and everyone onboard perished. By complete coincidence, the amateur wiring in WEC's building (another cost-saving measure by the administrator) shorted out on the same weekend, and the structure was reduced to ashes in a matter of hours. Fortunately, the practice's charts and appointment records were preserved in a back-up in the cloud. Unfortunately, no accounting records exist, nor does anyone know much about how many staff or doctors were employed in the practice, or the size and facilities of the now-lost office building.

Your team has been called in to restore WEC to its former glory. The practice saw 25,000 patient visits including postoperative and operated 1500 cataracts in the last 12 months.

Try this one yourself. The answers are found on page 212.

1. Name five priority actions you would take and why they are a priority.
2. Describe how many of each of these you will need:
    a. Exam rooms in the new office
    b. Total lay staff
    c. Number of receptionists, techs, surgical counselors, and billing staff
    d. Number of MDs and ODs
3. With this patient base, what would you expect annual net collections to be once the practice is restored?

Answers to questions on page 211.

1. Key activities are to preserve relationships with patients, have access to capital and get new providers on board. How about just selling the practice to a local competitor?
2. Expected numbers:
   a. 12 lanes
   b. ± 30 lay staff
   c. 6 receptionists, 12 techs, 1.5 surgical counselors, 3.8 to 4.0 billers
   d. A total of 4 DEs (eg, 4 MDs or 3 MDs and 2 ODs, or 2 MDs and 4 ODs)
3. Annual revenue of $4 to $5.5 million or so

CHAPTER 40

Right-Sizing Your Technical Department's Staffing Levels

Overhead will eat you alive if not constantly viewed as a parasite to be exterminated.
—Felix Dennis

The most expensive practice cost is lay staffing, at an average fully burdened cost today of about $45,000 per year. The most expensive segment of your lay team is your technicians, inclusive of work-up techs, scribes, and chairside assistants; special testing staff; back-office runners; and even those clerical staff who may be drafted to room patients or supervise the occasional visual field test.

This chapter will help you assess your own tech staffing levels.

To be able to compare one practice with another as we calculate the labor productivity of your technical staff, be sure to exclude any time they may be spending on surgical counseling, helping out at the front desk, or assisting with transcription. You should also omit any time they may spend on research studies or community outreach and screenings.

Wohl C, Pinto JB. *UP: Taking Ophthalmic Administrators and Their Management Teams to the Next Level of Skill, Performance, and Career Satisfaction, Second Edition* (pp 213-216).

Here's an easy starter calculation:

- Imagine you have a solo general ophthalmology practice.
- You see 550 patient visits* per month (a reasonable baseline goal in today's world).
- You employ a total of three techs working an average of 36 hours each per week.

The math is simple:

- By convention, we need to count total compensated work hours, whether regular time, overtime, paid sick leave, or vacation time. Typically, a full-time, 40-hour-per-week staffer will be paid for 2080 hours of work per year (40 hours × 52 weeks) or an average of 173 hours per month.
- In this sample practice, each tech is a 0.9 full-time equivalent (FTE). The three techs taken together add up to 2.7 FTEs.
- Multiplying 2.7 FTEs times 173 nominal hours in a month yields a total of 467 tech hours in the month.
- 467 hours divided by 550 visits boils down to 0.85 tech payroll hours per patient visit, or about 51 minutes.

What's normal? In this sample, general practice, liberal norms could be everything from 0.8 to 1.0 tech hour per patient visit.

It would be reasonable to be at the low end of this wide range if your doctors like to do relatively more of the patient work-up themselves, or if the practice is static, with the doctors nearing retirement, having fewer new patients to work up, and a desire to spare costs so they can top up their retirement savings.

At the other extreme, it might be reasonable to be at the high end of this normal range if your generalist doctors dislike routine work-up chores and choose to delegate as much of the exam as possible to highly trained technician staff—hopefully allowing them to see more patients.

Here are some other potential reasons for having a somewhat heavier tech staff:

- You have a young crew of only half-trained techs, who are not yet functioning fully.
- Your head tech is new and not yet managing the floor very efficiently; you and she have decided to keep the department somewhat overstaffed until she settles in.
- You have a high surgical density (as in a co-management–biased practice) and a significant percentage of your patients are surgical work-ups.
- The doctors have an assertive approach to testing and want patients to receive all such testing during the same visit.
- Your practice places a premium on concierge-level patient care, and you never want a patient left waiting for lack of a tech.
- You have a number of satellite offices, and techs travel routinely to several office locations throughout the week (resulting in some efficiency being lost to travel time).

---

*A note on patient visits. A patient visit, by convention, is a patient seen by a provider (an MD, DO, or OD professional). This includes compensated visits as well as uncompensated postoperative visits (when seen by a provider), and omits patients seen by a technician only (as for a pressure check or visual field exam). This metric omits surgical encounters. As a matter of routine, it does not count those few patients per month who may drop in for a minor clinic procedure with the doctor if they do not also receive an exam on that day, nor does it count the infrequent emergency department or admitted patient seen in the hospital. In a retinal practice, it should include injection visits.

The Influence of Subspecialty Care

Tech levels needed in your practice will vary markedly based on doctor subspecialty work. Pediatric and oculoplastic subspecialists, with lower patient volumes, can sometimes get by with only 0.6 tech hours per visit. Glaucoma subspecialists, especially those striving for higher production levels, are in line with generalists—about 0.8 to 1.0 hour per visit. Pure refractive surgeons will typically need 1.1 tech hours per patient visit to accommodate the extensive work-up demands of this subspecialty.

Retinal subspecialists need the most back-office support, with 1.3 tech hours per patient visit. This is driven by older/sicker/slower patients and by the extensive testing and treatment regimens in this subspecialty. Given the stronger economic productivity present in retina, the extra labor costs are rarely of any adverse consequence. Indeed, retinologists can typically get by spending around 25% of their cash flow on the full complement of lay labor, while generalists commonly spend 28% to 32%.

As a general observation, tech coverage levels in client general/anterior segment settings have been creeping upward with three factors: The rising number of visits seen in a day, the addition of special testing, and the increased use of scribes to accommodate to electronic health records.

If a doctor sees only 400 visits per month and can handle more of his own work-ups, then you may be fine with 0.6 to 0.7 tech hours per visit. As his monthly load grows to 500 visits or more, you will want the doctor to delegate more care, and he'll need proportionately more coverage so he can see more patients each day. The cost of adding one full-time technician is more than covered by adding two to three patients daily in clinic. In selected hypervolumetric settings (some general ophthalmologists are now stretching to 800 visits or more for one doctor per month), even more patient care and communication is delegated, so more tech time per patient is needed.

The addition of more special testing (nonmydriatic retinal cameras, dry eye testing, more aggressive optical coherence tomography testing, and the like) now has the average generalist client practice staffing at a level of 1.0 tech payroll hour per visit to be able to fit in all of the extra services and not run behind. Indeed, when we visit a practice and see lower levels of testing utilization (when compared to peers), the top driver is rarely physician circumspection or conservatism, but a lack of support staff, leading providers to simply say, "Well, we're kind of backed up today, let's just get that test the next time you're here in 6 months."

The increased use of chairside scribe-assistants is also escalating tech coverage levels. Two generations ago, vanguard doctors would use an assistant to room patients and perhaps take a basic history. Charts were kept on index cards. In the present environment, it's very fatiguing to be a provider trying to clear a full schedule without a scribe in the room.

At the same time that we're trying to push down labor costs, remember that ophthalmology is a largely fixed-cost profession. At typical net revenue yields per patient encounter, adding another tech is more than paid for by seeing just another two to three patients per day. If you're not scheduling a backlog of patients because of a lack of technical support, you should be adding, not subtracting, tech payroll hours.

Remember that every practice is different, and your practice owners get to create (and pay for) their own preferred environment. Some surgeons prefer a small, crack team of highly experienced and highly compensated techs. Others prefer to focus on raw headcounts and would rather employ a large number of low- to mid-level assistants. Fifteen techs at $25 per hour cost the same amount as 25 techs at $15 per hour. It's important to discuss staffing philosophies with your providers.

You may encounter an efficiency problem when you compress your clinic schedule into a few, intense hours each week, while paying for the same number of technical staff hours every day. This feast-or-famine approach is not only tough on the economics of the practice (especially if you staff for peak patient hours) but can also harm morale and frustrate providers and patients alike. You have two solutions to apply: Either spread patients out more evenly through the week, which can also result in more efficient facility utilization, or keep the intense sessions, sending staff home during down times.

Interestingly, technical staffing efficiency does not increase with group size. Indeed, if you're not cautious, doctors in a large group practice can start competing with each other to build their own staff empires. To overcome this, some group practices directly charge each owner for his or her technical support staff. When this transition is made, overstaffed departments become leaner almost overnight as each surgeon begins to rationally meter down personal needs instead of empire building.

• • •

Now is the time to develop a more robust understanding of practice labor costs. Every expected trend for eye care—as demand soars and physician cohorts shrink—will lead to a continued substitution of labor. It may be hard to fathom today, but the year will come when paraprofessionals (and computers) will not only room and work up a patient for you, but also generate a suggested diagnosis, course of treatment, and return interval for you to approve or revise. It's coming fast. Don't blink.

CHAPTER 41

Reducing Practice Labor Costs by Measuring and Improving Staff Turnover and Separation Rates

Beware of little expenses.
A small leak will sink a great ship.
—Benjamin Franklin

Price doesn't make deals,
and salary doesn't control your career.
—Christopher Voss

Support staff are the largest single cost of operating an ophthalmology practice. The typical general/geriatric practice spends about 30 cents out of every dollar it takes in for receptionists, techs, billers, managers, and all the rest. This figure has climbed for a generation and will keep climbing with inflation. Even with the lowest rates of inflation (official US government policy is to induce a 2% annual inflation rate), wage rates for quality workers will inexorably rise, as revenue per unit of patient service continues to stagnate (and even fall sharply for our clients in Canada).

Unfortunately, as in almost every service sector business, it's still difficult for eye care practices to drive greater labor efficiencies. Until especially charming robot staff are invented, your customers will need an irreducible level of human

Wohl C, Pinto JB. *UP: Taking Ophthalmic Administrators and Their Management Teams to the Next Level of Skill, Performance, and Career Satisfaction, Second Edition* (pp 217-219). © 2021 Taylor & Francis Group.

contact with your organization. So, it is becoming more critical in a fixed and falling fee environment to keep a ceiling on staffing costs in other ways.

Staffing expenses can get out of control for a number of reasons, including:

- Overstaffing, if you miscalculate your labor requirements
- Poor recruitment and selection, if you are inattentive in hiring
- Poor skills development, if you underinvest in training
- Poor staff productivity, if you don't adequately supervise your staff
- Excessive rates of pay, caused by naïve or intentional generosity, or a misunderstanding of local labor rates

A helpful way to assess staffing dynamics is to look at average tenure. This is simply derived. Start with a list of all current staff, showing their dates of hire. For each member of your team, calculate the number of years employed. For example, a tech employed the last 70 months has been in your practice for 5.8 years. Add up all of the resulting years-in-service, divide by the number of staffers, and you will get the average tenure. In older, well-managed client practices, those making wise hiring decisions, this average figure can be in excess of 8 years. In practices with high turnover rates, the average tenure may be no more than 1 or 2 years.

What's the cost to your practice of insufficient tenure, excessive turnover, and separation rates? The American Management Association estimated that turnover costs range from 25% to almost 200% of annual compensation depending on the job function. Using the low 25% figure and applying this to the typical $45,000 fully burdened, cost per practice staffer yields a cost of more than $11,000 every time you lose a staff member.

There are numerous direct and indirect drivers of this:

- Severance and unemployment benefits costs
- Impacts on the morale of remaining staff
- Lost provider productivity when technical staff are lost
- The lost contacts and knowledge of departing staff
- Advertising, agency fees, and background checks for recruitment and vetting
- The overtime costs and lost productivity in other job functions of fill-in staff
- Transient drops in the quality of customer service, leading to some unhappy, even lost, patients
- The time of management staff and co-workers to select and train the new worker

Obviously, it's unacceptably expensive to run a practice with excessive turnover rates. Now that you understand a few ways of measuring turnover and retention, let's discuss what can you do as a practice owner or executive to improve the numbers.

The largest corporations in the United States have tighter hiring practices than the typical ophthalmologist. They have formal employee retention programs, monitor employee satisfaction, and invest in programs to reward their best people. Proportionately more modest (but similarly effective) tactics are reasonable to adopt in eye care, especially as demands grow for experienced health care workers and low unemployment rates in most markets make it difficult to find talented trainees. There are hundreds of simple tactics used by practices where we find the lowest turnover rates. Here are just a few:

- Using real-world, skills-based preemployment tests to ensure that workers have demonstrated an aptitude for the specific job being filled.
- Only making a new hire after every potential co-worker of the new employee has interviewed the final candidates.
- Understanding the early career history of your potential hire. Staff who started working in their early teens seem to make the best workers.
- Understanding the motivation level of your candidate employees. Is it strong enough to stay the course on the difficult days?
- Making sure that all doctor–staff interaction is positive and supportive. The highest turnover rates are not found in practices with low wages but in practices where adverse doctor behavior saps morale.
- Expressing appreciation often and publicly.
- Using surprise bonuses judiciously to reward exceptional performance.
- Being strategically intimate with staff. Sharing your dreams for the practice, so they have a context for coming in and doing their best each morning.
- Fostering staff-to-staff relationships. Occasional after-hours group socializing, paid for by the practice, helps to connect staff with each other. Hiring the friends of existing staff can be an effective way to bond both parties to the company.

Savvy managers and owners realize they are not only competing with other eye practices but with the entire local employer base for the best workers. Just as it's easier to retain a patient than find a new one, it's much more cost-effective to retain the staff you have than to be stuck on an unnecessary, expensive hiring treadmill.

CHAPTER 42

Unpolished Clinic Operations?

Examine and Smooth Your Patient Flow With This Daily Clinic Review Tool

If you do not change direction,
you may end up where you are heading.
—Lao Tzu

Don't be afraid to show your vulnerability.
Be transparent with your team,
even when the truth may be unpopular or inconvenient.
—Bill George

We met recently for a board and senior management staff retreat to discuss practice operations, including a number of opportunities to improve clinical flow and efficiency.

By the mid-point of the meeting, having heard doctor after doctor complain about continued inefficiencies on the clinic floor, it was obvious they had never really provided much in the way of cohesive feedback to their managers about what was so vexing. As one manager posed, "Why haven't you said something to us before this?"

What then resulted was a brainstorm to formalize the feedback process: "Let's provide a fast, simple way for doctors, at the end of a clinic day, to let their managers know just how they think things went that day."

Wohl C, Pinto JB. *UP: Taking Ophthalmic Administrators and Their Management Teams to the Next Level of Skill, Performance, and Career Satisfaction, Second Edition* (pp 221-224).

The following is a reporting and feedback tool to help get you organized and help providers communicate their frustrations and needs more effectively.

Daily Clinic Review Tool

Office location: ______________________________

Doctor: ______________________________

Date: ______________________________

a.m. __________ **p.m.** __________ **Both:** ______________

Instructions: One of the missing links in clinic management is an effective feedback tool to provide doctors and managers with a common starting point for evaluating and improving weak areas. Too often, doctors will confront managers about events from the distant past, or unfairly amplify one small error in an otherwise great day. This review tool can help foster the communication needed to agree on, make, and then monitor needed improvements.

1. Pick a reasonable clinic review interval. This might be daily if your center has large, ongoing difficulties, or as infrequently as once every few months (in the spirit of basic housekeeping) if the practice generally runs very well.
2. At the end of every monitored clinic day (or half day, if that's the length of a work day), give each participating provider a copy of this review form to be completed before leaving for the day.
3. When the form is completed, it's handed to the head tech for supplemental comments, and then to the site manager or administrator for their written input as well. Such comments could include notes about the day's staffing levels, doctor arrival time, an excessive number of work-in or no-show patients, broken equipment, etc.
4. The efficiency calculations at the end of this tool are then completed by the administrator or a designated staffer.
5. Conduct periodic group meetings (with doctors, technicians, and managers present) to review the completed forms, compare impressions, come up with needed improvements, and check for progress.

Provider to Complete

Please rate on a 1 to 10 scale (1 = low/poor, 10 = high/excellent) the following aspects of today's clinic:

____ Physical plant. Clean, supplies on hand, equipment in good repair, temperature, etc.

____ Clinic running on time. Not running late.

____ Effectiveness and utilization of the patient scheduling template.

____ Overall competency and tempo of the entire practice team (both front and back).

____ Completeness of patient records.

____ Competency, accuracy, and tempo of the technicians, scribes, and special testing staff.

____ Your sense that the head tech and/or site manager was on top of clinic flow and tempo.

____ Flexibility of the team. Did we adjust to the ebb and flow of patient volumes?

____ Other: ____

Please write down at least two specific ideas for how we could have improved today's clinic:

1. ____

2. ____

Head Tech Comments:

Site Manager/Administrator Comments:

Daily Efficiency Calculations

A. Total hours worked: ____

(eg, If the clinic opened with first appointments at 8:00 a.m., worked through lunch, and discharged the last patient at 6:15 p.m., that's 10.25 hours.)

B. Total patients seen: ____

(Count encounters as a patient seen by a physician or optometrist; don't overcount, as by counting special testing events as separate encounters and don't undercount by omitting postoperative visits.)

C. Patients per doctor hour (divide "B" by "A"): ____

(There is no one right number for this ratio. It could be nine or more patients per hour in a highly efficient, mature cataract practice with a large percentage of postoperative patients, or as few as two or three patients per hour in a subspecialty practice. It's helpful to develop your own internal benchmarks.)

D. Number of exam rooms used: ____

(Count active, fully equipped, doctor rooms only; omit special testing, procedure, and tech-only work-up rooms.)

E. Exam room hours (multiply "A" times "D"): ____

(eg, If you have four exam rooms, and 8.5 hours of active operation, that's 34 exam room hours.)

F. Patient visits per exam room hour (Divide "B" by "E"): ____

(When averaged out over an entire month or year, this benchmark in a general/geriatric eye clinic is typically 0.8 to 1.2 patient visits per exam room hour. Looking at this metric just one day at a time can result in a somewhat higher or lower number. Again, it's important to internally benchmark these figures for your own special situation, and look at the results over time.)

G. Number of clinical support staff used: ____

(Be sure to count all lay workers who act as technicians, scribes, or special testing staff. If your practice uses optometrists as "super-techs" or refractionists, rather than independent providers of patient care, then include such doctors as part of the lay staff in your calculations.)

H. Total techs/scribes/testing staff payroll hours (multiply "A" times "G"): ____

(You'll obviously need to do some individual calculating if not all clinical staff work the same number of hours in a day.)

I. Techs/scribes/testing staff payroll hours per patient visit (divide "H" by "B"): ____

(As with the patient visits per exam room hour measurement in F, when averaged out over an entire month or year, this benchmark in a general/geriatric eye clinic with one location is typically 0.8 to 1.0. Looking at this metric just one day at a time can result in a somewhat higher or lower figure.)

CHAPTER 43

How a Pro Forma Helps You See the Future

It does not do to leave a live dragon out of your calculations, if you live near him.
—J.R.R. Tolkien, *The Hobbit*

Someone's sitting in the shade today because someone planted a tree a long time ago.
—Warren Buffett

By failing to prepare, you are preparing to fail.
—Benjamin Franklin

Ophthalmic practices have thousands of moving parts. Thoughtful, intentional, and, especially, documented decision making is key to keeping the practice machine well oiled.

There are numerous "oil cans."

One is to develop and follow a written strategic plan. Fewer than 10% of ophthalmic practices have a formal, written strategic plan. Decisions impacting the practice's future are often made opportunistically, rather than by developing and following a written, regularly updated plan with an appropriate time horizon. This may be as little as 2 to 3 years or stretch to a decade or longer.

Another disciplined oil can for your practice, one that is often embedded within a strategic plan, is called a *pro forma*.

Wohl C, Pinto JB. *UP: Taking Ophthalmic Administrators and Their Management Teams to the Next Level of Skill, Performance, and Career Satisfaction, Second Edition* (pp 225-228). © 2021 Taylor & Francis Group.

A pro forma is a financial spreadsheet, of greater or lesser detail and complexity, that can help you predict the outcome of any proposed business activity. A pro forma can help you assess:

- The financial impact of adding a new provider to the practice
- The likely result of adding a new service like elective plastics or hearing aids
- How you will be impacted by the imminent retirement of a partner
- Whether it makes sense to merge with another practice
- If it would be better to keep or abandon a faltering satellite office
- The impact of taking on more office space in your next lease contract

With or without a strategic plan, a detailed pro forma can be a useful guide that helps owners and administrators move beyond gut hunches and project more closely the potential impact of your practice's prospective actions.

As a very simple example, let's say you are the administrator for a solo practitioner, Dr. Smith. You are considering the addition of an optometrist. You are also planning to expand your office somewhat by adding a couple of exam rooms.

A pro forma is only as good as the underlying assumptions you use to develop it. And although your initial assumptions are often imperfect, working through this process shows you how the moving parts fit or don't fit together.

The following is a sample pro forma for Dr. Smith that can be used to project the possible outcomes of actions he is considering. This sample is a <u>very</u> basic illustration and probably will be less elaborate than the much more complex pro formas you are likely to employ.

Dr. Smith's Basic Pro Forma Review: What Will Be the Impact on My Solo Practice of Adding a Full-Time Optometrist?

	Dr. Smith's Current Annual Economics	Projected Economics After Adding an Optometrist
Baseline collections	$1,100,000	$1,100,000
Added OD professional fee collections		$400,000
Added OD optical collections		$175,000
Total collections	**$1,100,000**	**$1,675,000**
Baseline practice expenses	$715,000	$715,000
Incremental OD wages, taxes, and benefits		$150,000
Incremental OD general and administrative support		$200,000
Incremental optical expenses		$105,000
Total Expenses	**$715,000**	**$1,170,000**
Total profit available for the MD-owner	**$385,000**	**$505,000**

Assumptions:

- Current practice has $1.1 million in collections and $715,000 in expenses.
- After an initial transition period, MD revenue production will remain the same.
- OD will work full time (40 hours per week).
- OD will be paid a total of $150,000 in wages, taxes, and benefits.
- OD will see 350 visits per month with an average professional fee ticket of about $95 per visit.
- OD will contribute $175,000 per year in optical collections.
- Optical goods and labor overhead margin on the incremental sales will be 60%.
- OD will require two techs, two additional clerical support staff, and also $40,000 annually in general and administrative support and in amortizing capital outlays, to add two exam rooms.
- Practice has a backlog of patients and will relatively quickly fill up the new doctor's schedule.

As you can see from this simple example, if the underlying assumptions are correct, Dr. Smith stands to enjoy a 31% pay raise if he adds an optometrist. Of course, it could take a year or longer to achieve the ultimate financial result in the right-hand column. For a few quarters, Dr. Smith may actually take a pay cut, because of revenue lags caused by credentialing delays and gradual patient volume growth, and the usual front-end expenses of any expansion like this.

In order to understand how cash flow may change over time with even a simple practice project like adding a single provider, you can expand your pro forma to show not just the end-point result, but the intermediate collections, expenses, and profits as well. For a very long cycle project, like opening satellites or a merger event, you may need to expand the month-by-month or quarter-by-quarter projection out to a year or longer.

Simplifying greatly, this would look something like:

	Year 1				Year 2	
	Quarter 1	*Quarter 2*	*Quarter 3*	*Quarter 4*	*Quarter 1*	*Quarter 2*
Collections	300,000	330,000	363,000	399,000	439,000	483,000
Expenses	200,000	270,000	250,000	270,000	300,000	330,000
Profit	100,000	60,000	113,000	129,000	139,000	153,000

Until you are comfortable with this tool, and for large impact decisions, have your accountant and other advisors work with you to tighten and expand the set of underlying assumptions.

And here's a last thought. At this point, you might notice that these pro formas, even though they are materially simplified, look a lot like an annual budget. And of course that's what an annual budget is—merely a forecast (like the simple example for Dr. Smith) of what's going to happen in the future.

Only a minority of practices generate an overall pro forma budget each year, and then use this as a disciplined comparison to actual performance. And many practices that try annual budgeting abandon the exercise because so much can change in a year. But even if you don't formally budget, the next time a large project surfaces, try to create a pro forma spreadsheet. As the saying goes, "Gather the facts, and let the facts make the decision for you."

CHAPTER 44

Being an Effective Steward of Practice Resources

Conducting "Rounds" on Your Practice's Support Systems

Genius is 1% inspiration and 99% perspiration.
—Thomas Edison

I told the doctor I broke my leg in two places.
He told me to quit going to those places.
—Henny Youngman

A prominent learning aid for physicians has always been "rounding" patients in a hospital.

Individually or in small groups, the doctor goes go from one patient bed to the next, checking progress, sharing a laugh if time permitted, scanning the latest vital signs, and ordering new tests, all under the watchful eye of doctor superiors.

Such case-based learning is grueling, and occasionally embarrassing, but effective. And it is the basis for many nonmedical graduate programs, including business and finance degrees.

Even today, the most clinically successful practices we know approach each patient as another opportunity for medical learning.

Wohl C, Pinto JB. *UP: Taking Ophthalmic Administrators and Their Management Teams to the Next Level of Skill, Performance, and Career Satisfaction, Second Edition* (pp 229-232). © 2021 Taylor & Francis Group.

What we've observed in our fieldwork is that the most financially successful managers also apply the same intellectual curiosity to their administrative rounds.

How can you get your practice started with this or enhance what you already do with this approach? Doctors in training memorize various question sets to ask each patient, depending on their presenting condition. With experience, the clinical question set expands; some questions are skipped and others added. You can do the same thing as an administrator or department head. We present here a starter set of questions you can apply in the various business domains of your practice.

Clinical Services

- Are we conducting enough tech training of high enough quality to have everyone on the team up to speed? (Shoot for no less than 2 hours of training per month.)
- What is our current ratio of back office staff to patient visit? (Count the total number of tech, scribe, and testing payroll hours in a month and divide by the number of total patient visits, including postoperative visits: the normal figure is about 1 staff hour per visit in general care, and up to 1.3 hours in subspecialty care.)
- Has sufficient cross-training occurred to allow techs to scribe or scribes to do testing, so that the team is more flexible and can flow during the clinic day to where they are most needed?
- Is any equipment out of repair or in need of replacement?

Billing and Patient Accounts

- What is the cycle time now between seeing a patient in the clinic, posting their charge, and submitting a claim? (You want to hear that it's taking no more than 24 hours to post and another 24 hours to submit. Less is always better.)
- Looking at our aging report, what percentage of our open accounts are out over 9
- 0 days? (Under 12% is desirable; under 8% is seen in superior departments.)
- What is our claims denial rate? What is the most common cause of a denial? Are we working our denials actively?
- Are we on top of refunds, or have we allowed these payable amounts to creep up?

Reception and Call Center Management

- What percentage of our desired template are we filling? (If you have the capacity and desire to see 40 patients per day, you should have 42 appointment slots, allowing for the typical 5% no-show rate.)
- What is the average primary waiting time now? (That's the time passing between the patient's actual appointment time and when they are first roomed by a staffer. It should be under 20 minutes in most settings.)

- When is the next available nonemergency appointment? (It should ideally be 3 weeks out or sooner.)
- What do our phone reports tell us about how diligent we are in answering the phone promptly and not letting callers roll over to voicemail?

Facilities Management

- Is there one, single person (typically the practice administrator) who is responsible for the condition of our office facilities? Does this person impose high enough standards?
- Are our facilities slowly degrading, staying about the same, or improving?
- Are building maintenance, cleaning, painting, and gardening vendors staying on top of their respective jobs?
- Is the quality of our facilities in line with the image we want to project? (Or are we trying to sell premium/elective services in an office that does not reflect that?)

Marketing and Development

- Do we have a written marketing plan and goals this year for things like new patients, cataract cases, and number of referring doctors? Are we on track with these goals?
- What have we done this month to ascertain patient or referral source satisfaction? What were the results?
- Have we written thank you notes to patients who referred to us this month?
- Have we audited recall work to ensure that each doctor's return-to-clinic order has resulted in an appointment being made?

Human Resources

- Are we following all applicable state and federal employment laws?
- Are all staff performance reviews up to date? Are personnel files updated after every review?
- Is the employee policy manual current and being followed?
- Are we treating everyone fairly, or are we overlooking adverse behaviors in selected staff because they are otherwise exceptionally skilled or being protected from criticism by their doctor?
- When was the last time we assessed staff satisfaction and what were the results?

Bookkeeping and Accounting

- Are our vendors being paid in an appropriate time frame?
- Are invoices checked against purchase orders?
- Does a partner-level physician sign off on checks? (Note that this commonly shifts to a nonphysician in larger practices.)
- Are financial reports available shortly after the end of each month? (The standard used to be 20 days and now is 10 days or less.)
- Do we have access to adequate capital reserves? (Adding up recoverable accounts receivable, bank accounts, and credit lines, you should have ready access to 3 or more months of average practice expenses before nominal physician compensation.)

Financial Performance

- What's our year-to-date profit margin? (This can be wide-ranging, from 30% to 50% or more, and still be normal for a given practice. It's important to track your trend line and compare to norms for your kind of practice.)
- What percentage of cash flow are we spending on lay support staff? Facilities? (Answers should come in at about 30% and 5%, respectively.)
- What are the average collections per patient visit this month, and are we trending up or down? ($150 to $225 or more is commonly seen.)

Optical Performance

- What are our optical collections per patient visit? (This can range widely from $15 to $65.)
- Do we have the right number of opticians? (The acceptable figure is $20,000 or more in annual optical collections per dispensing optician.)
- What's the recent cost of goods sold (COGS) figure? (The COGS ratio, which is simply the total frame and lens vendor costs divided by total optical collections, ranges between 30% and 40% in most settings.)

• • •

How often should you perform your administrative rounds? About once a month is sufficient, but just like in medicine, frail practices require a more frequent and vigilant approach. In the most stable and secure practices, once a quarter may be fine.

CHAPTER 45

A New Benchmark ORUS

Your Ophthalmic Resource Utilization Score

Efficiency is doing things right;
effectiveness is doing the right things.
—Peter Drucker

There can be economy only where there is efficiency.
—Benjamin Disraeli

The most dangerous kind of waste is
the waste we don't recognize.
—Shigeo Shingo

As the administrator of your practice, the first line of your job description could read: "Resource Allocation Authority." This may sound fancy, but as you're about to read, it's really the most basic part of your job as an administrator or senior department head.

In these leadership roles, what resources do you have at your command to serve your patients?

- Providers
- Lay staff
- Clinical and surgical facilities
- Technology
- Reputation

Wohl C, Pinto JB. *UP: Taking Ophthalmic Administrators and Their Management Teams to the Next Level of Skill, Performance, and Career Satisfaction, Second Edition* (pp 233-236).

- Relationships
- Internal and external expertise
- And, finally, time (which is always fleeting)

In years past, an ophthalmic leader could leave a lot of potential resources lying fallow, because profit margins were so high. A generation ago, when one could easily bring 50% to the bottom line in an anterior segment practice, few really cared if there was an extra staffer up at the front desk, or if someone ordered so many extra medical supplies that a few of them went out of date before they could be used.

In the present and future environment, that is all changed. You not only need to think coarsely in terms of "Do we have an extra worker we don't really need?" but more granularly, "Can I send Mary home an hour early and bring $20 to the bottom line?"

As a practice manager, you may relish this granular accountability. Indeed, if you came from tighter sectors of the economy—retail or restaurants or hospitality—you're probably saying, "What took ophthalmology so long to catch up?"

Most of you reading this are probably already benchmarking at least a few key indicators and perhaps even a slew of them. These should be shared with your physician or board every month or quarter. Here's a possible augmentation to the benchmarking you already perform, a gross, composite score of what percentage of your key resources of your current resources you are actually using. This is a simple, fast way to objectively answer the question: "Are we doing all that we can with all that we have?"

There are just three segments to this composite Ophthalmic Resources Utilization Score (ORUS): providers, lay staff, and facilities. Taken together, these three segments are not only the most important, they are also the costliest, consuming a majority of every dollar you collect. All three of these segments are couched in terms of what percentage of the maximum patient throughput each is achieving.

Provider Utilization Segment

Every ophthalmologist and optometrist has his or her own personal capacity to see patients. We have physician clients who personally see more than 1000 visits per month. And others who gasp at any more than 350 visits. How many patients you can see depends on a number of factors, but can be reduced to this simple recap:

- A general/geriatric or corneal ophthalmic provider is at 100% of nominal full capacity at 550 visits (including postoperative visits; not including surgery or tech-only visits) per month.
- A retinal, glaucoma, or pediatric physician provider is at 100% at 450 visits per month.
- A plastics subspecialist will comfortably see 350 visits per month.
- An optometrist in the typical mid-level provider role can comfortably see 350 visits per month; although with tech support more typically allotted to physicians, there are ODs who thrive in this environment seeing 450 to 500 visits per month.

Let's say your practice has one general ophthalmologist, one retinal specialist, and two ODs, named Smith, Jones, Davis, and Edwards, respectively. Make a table like this:

Doctor	Average Monthly Patient Visits	Typical Potential Monthly Patient Visits
Smith	500	550
Jones	375	450
Davis	450	350
Edwards	275	350
Total	**1600**	**1700**

Next, you can simply calculate what percent of nominal capacity your providers are achieving as a cohort by dividing their actual volume (1600) by their potential volume (1700) to get 94%.

Lay Staff Utilization Segment

There are several ways to measure lay staff efficiency. These include:

- Overall lay staff payroll hours per patient visit
- Tech, reception, or billing staff (broken out by department) per visit
- Staffing costs as a percentage of collections
- Annual collections per full-time equivalent (FTE) staffer in the practice

For the purpose of this ORUS scoring system, we use the number of overall lay staff hours per patient visit as a proxy for overall lay staffing efficiency. You can calculate this simply. Determine the average monthly core lay staff payroll hours the practice pays for—this can be readily determined from most payroll report forms. Omit ambulatory surgical center, optical, and contact lens staff. Divide the resulting hours by the average monthly patient visits in your practice.

In eye care, the high-water mark for this metric in all general and subspecialty settings is 3.0 lay staff hours per patient visit—any higher and you are probably drowning in staff. A reasonable performance target in all segments except retina is 2.5 hours. In a pure retina practice, 2.8 hours is the target. (It's interesting to know that it takes Toyota about 30 staff hours to build a whole car.)

So let's imagine our sample practice with four providers and 1600 visits per month has 4750 lay staff payroll hours per month. That would be just over 27 staffers. What's their efficiency score for this segment? Simple. First divide 4750 lay staff hours by 1600 visits to get 3.0 staff hours per visit, which sounds a tad overstaffed, even when you consider that this is a mixed general-retinal practice that can reasonably use a bit more staff support than a general practice. All the same, we should be aiming to cover the practice well with no more than 2.7 lay hours per visit. So we can make following calculation to get the staffing efficiency percentage:

- With 4750 staff hours, they should be able to see 1759 patients per month (4750/2.7 = 1759).
- But they actually only see 1600 visits.
- So, we divide 1600 by 1759 and get an efficiency percentage of 91%.

Facility Utilization Segment

Last, we calculate facility utilization. How should that be done? Again, we resort to indexing patient visits—this time the relationship between the number of exam rooms and the number of examinations.

In the typical, efficient general practice it takes 1 room hour to transit a patient visit. A practice like the one we are using as an example here, with 1600 visits per month, requires 9.2 exam rooms (1600 visits per month divided by 173 hours in the average month).

But imagine that Smith & Jones Eye actually has 12 exam rooms. How many room-hours do they have? And how do we calculate their utilization rate? Simple: 12 exam rooms times 173 hours in the average month makes for 2076 room hours. And they really only need 1600 room hours. So we divide 1600 by 2076 and get 77%. (Note: There is not enough facility utilization difference between general practices and subspecialty practices to worry about. We simply use the metric of 1 exam room hour being needed per visit.)

The composite score in this example of Smith & Jones Eye is the average of the three utilization scores:

(94% + 91% + 77%)/3 = 87%

Said another way, Smith & Jones Eye is working at about 87% of its overall potential capacity. What should they be at? That's entirely up to Smith & Jones, of course. But speaking economically, practice profitability improves the closer you can get to 100%.

Try this ORUS out in your own practice. If your score is lower than you would like, you have two options to improve—shed costly unused capacity or boost patient visits.

CHAPTER 46

Improving Your No-Show Rate

Lost time is never found again.
—Benjamin Franklin

Filling 100% of your desired appointment slots daily is a top goal and priority found in the best-run practices. No-show patients must be kept to a minimum for the sake of both your patients and your bottom line. Underbooked appointment templates and excessive no-show rates cost the practice significant revenue and keep patients from needed care.

The following are the challenges of this multifaceted problem and success factors to control the rate. First, some facts:

- Normal no-show rates for anterior segment practices are 5% in most settings, edging up to 6% to 8% in coastal/urban settings.

Wohl C, Pinto JB. *UP: Taking Ophthalmic Administrators and Their Management Teams to the Next Level of Skill, Performance, and Career Satisfaction, Second Edition* (pp 237-239).

- In the rural United States and in retinal practices, norms are generally 2% to 4%.
- Pediatric practices and optometrists are typically in the 10% to 20% range.

To calculate your no-show rate, divide the number of daily no-show appointments by the number of scheduled appointments you had when the day began. Be sure your reports are showing only true no-shows and not rescheduled appointments. A patient who was expected in the office this morning, but who calls (even at the last minute) to reschedule, is not a no-show, by way of convention.

Track all no-shows in your electronic health record system. Be sure to follow up with a phone call the same day to reschedule the appointment. Ideally, we recommend calling within 1 hour of the missed appointment, which often allows the patient to be squeezed back into the schedule on the same day. Note this action in the patient chart.

Once the data are collected, analyzing it by doctor, location, and the day of the week (and even time of day if you are tracking a severe problem) will provide the patterns you need to deduce the cause and reduce the rate. You may also find that the average is different from doctor to doctor in the same practice. For example, surgically oriented and senior doctors typically have lower no-show rates than younger doctors with a less-bonded patient base.

There are many common drivers for excessive no-show rates:

- Higher no-show rates are most generally due to doctor-mediated gaps (eg, a failure to impress on the patient the importance of keeping the next appointment because of family history).
- Sometimes excess no-shows can be due to lower levels of patient satisfaction. Patient: "Sure I'll make an appointment..." ("because you are insisting, but I'm not actually going to come in because I don't like it here").
- Some of the problem is due to clerical gaps. It is common to see staff insisting that they "really, really" make reminder calls, but when you audit formally, you find that some or all of the calls are missing. You can't just take staff at their word that they are making the calls, you need to audit directly.
- If you are booking appointments out for 1 year, which is recommended, build a system that reminds the patient earlier than the typical 2 days in advance. We commonly advise a reminder via phone call, text, or email set 1 to 2 weeks in advance and then another 2 days ahead of the appointment. The more last-minute the reminder is, the higher the chance of a forgotten appointment.
- Pediatric and higher-volume Medicaid practices tend to have much higher no-show rates. A common workaround for this is to multiply the number of appointment reminders, for example, automated calls 5 days out, live calls 3 days out to those who did not respond to the auto-calls, then a final automated call 1 day out to everyone. This obviously mildly irritates the diligent patient, but often accomplishes the desired result of a lower no-show rate.

Here are a few common approaches to mitigate an excessively high rate:

- If your practice is in high demand, keep a call list ready for patients available on short notice to fill empty appointment slots.
- Schedule the repeat offenders at times when it will affect the overall schedule the least (eg, at the end of the clinic schedule).

- Write a policy to discharge patients who are persistent no-shows. Provide appropriate notice for them to find an alternate doctor.
- Don't book more than two family member visits at a time, unless you purposely make an exception for a family with whom you are familiar. This avoids a larger gap in the schedule if they are all no-shows.
- If your systems allow, find the best reminder method for each patient, (eg, automated text, email, phone call, or postcard reminders). In purely geriatric practices, no-show rates may come down if you experiment with live calls rather than automated calls. We have seen settings where the no-show rate drops in half when a shift is made from auto-calls to live calls.
- Consider charging a no-show fee of $25 to $50 and waive the fee liberally to avoid ill will. This was first tried in pediatrics and is now seen in perhaps 10% of practices overall. Some practices now keep a credit card on file to facilitate such charges, just as we now commonly see in hotels and restaurants.
- Establish enough appointment slots so that based on your average no-show rates you will usually have a full clinic every day (and live with the fact that sometimes the no-show rate will be much lower, creating a stressful day).
- Conduct a periodic recall audit. Pick 10 patient visits at random from the past week. Note the patient number, age, payer, principal diagnosis, the doctor's return-to-clinic order, and whether an appointment or recall was made at checkout. In an average client practice, we see at least a 10% error rate (eg, wrong return-to-clinic order, no appointment made) until the practice turns its attention to the responsible protocol gaps. This simple audit has two benefits: It will discover continuity of care gaps that you may not have noticed, and it will help keep staff and providers on their toes, knowing that a spot check is being made.

• • •

Three final tips:

1. Patient satisfaction is a key driver for improving no-show rates. Strong, bonded relationships between doctors (and staff) and patients help reduce the number of no-shows.
2. No-show rates can accelerate quickly when not being monitored regularly. Generate a report at least monthly to keep close tabs on any internal changes that may happen subtly.
3. Make a reduction in no-show rates a priority for your managers and staff. Remind managers that avoiding just one missed appointment a day can cover the annual salary for a receptionist or technician.

Section VII

Leading Together With the Doctors in Your Practice

CHAPTER 47

Practice Business Problems?

Think Like a Doctor

Success is almost totally dependent upon drive and persistence. The extra energy required to make another effort or try another approach is the secret of winning.

—Denis Waitley

Whether you are an administrator, mid-level manager, or doctor, here is what the smartest administrators and doctors recognized years ago: To solve a business problem in your practice, simply start thinking like a physician.

Doctors have unwittingly been trained to manage business problems effectively, but they may need your help to realize how to apply their knowledge.

Here's what we mean. An ophthalmologist sees a patient who presents with one of the objective signs of suspected glaucoma—elevated intraocular pressure. She knows what the pressure is supposed to be, and knows additional signs to look for and tests to apply. She also has a variety of proven medicines and surgical

Wohl C, Pinto JB. *UP: Taking Ophthalmic Administrators and Their Management Teams to the Next Level of Skill, Performance, and Career Satisfaction, Second Edition* (pp 243-248). © 2021 Taylor & Francis Group.

interventions as options to treat the patient's disease. She chooses one or more of these interventions, measures the positive results, and then monitors for adverse signs and symptoms on subsequent clinic visits.

Boiled down, that's how simple ophthalmic practice management can really be—discover suspected problems, verify your suspicions with objective measurements, apply proven treatments, confirm improvements, and monitor for any regression.

When you are challenged by department managers or physicians who want to jump to action prior to following these five steps, remind them of this proven way to problem solve. It's hiding in plain sight in every medical practice

Here are a few practical examples of this step-wise approach to management in practices large and small.

Are Our Staffing Costs Excessive?

If you think about it, excessive lay labor costs are a kind of business "disease," sapping your enterprise of free cash flow that could be better invested in expanding patient services, upgrading technology, improving facilities, or even giving the doctors a well-deserved pay raise. If it had a fancy medical name, this business management disease might be called "hyperstaffemia."

If you were thinking like a doctor and suspecting you were overstaffed, what would you do next? Lab tests! In this case, the tests and normative values for practice health are pretty well established. Here are some examples:

- Fully burdened lay staffing costs (wages, taxes, benefits) in most cases should be at or under 32% of collections.
- Your practice should be generating $10,000 per month or more in collections per lay staff full-time equivalent (FTE; one staff member working 40 hours per week).
- If you add up all the technician, scribe, and special testing staff payroll hours in a year, the resulting figure should be equal to or less than the number of total patient visits your practice generates in a year (for a general practice and 10% to 30% higher for an all-retina or LASIK practice).
- Your dispensing optical staff should be generating $200,000 or more each in annual sales.

If one or more of these lab values are out of normal ranges, apply the needed medicine, such as cutting back hours or reducing positions. Like any good administrator or clinician, don't act on your instincts alone, but call on the counsel of your fellow managers in the practice or seek outside help. Once the numbers look right again, monitor overall productivity monthly on a graph showing patient visits vs total staff payroll hours or staffing costs as a percent of revenue.

Should We Close Our Faltering Part-Time Satellite Office?

Let's have some fun and call this practice management disease "officemia," a very common malady in practices that at times overreach. The differential diagnosis is easy, and the test is painless.

For each office location, including your main office, calculate the average monthly collections over the past year or so. Then calculate the average monthly expenses (with the most accurate by-location cost allocations you can muster) and derive average monthly profit by location. Divide the average monthly profit for each location by the number of physician hours spent in each location. For example, if your satellite office generates average monthly profits of $15,000 and your various doctors spend a total of 125 hours per month in this location (inclusive of travel time) then the average profit per doctor hour is only about $120, which may be a little on the light side compared to other locations. (For a healthy practice, you should be generating $150 or more in profit per doctor hour; surgically dense practices hit $500 or more.)

The treatment plan for officemia involves one of two practical care pathways. Either act to increase the profit per doctor hour in a faltering location or close the satellite office down. You may be able to increase profits per hour in a number of ways, such as billing more effectively, seeing more patients, if they are available, spending less time in the office, or marketing to increase the surgical and revenue yield per patient visit. Before closing any one satellite office, you should ask two critical questions:

1. Have we done everything we reasonably could to improve the performance of this office?
2. Will the freed-up doctor time be applied more usefully in another office?

Our Office Staff Seem to Be Agitated. Turnover Is Excessive. What Should We Do?

We are going to call this one "teamitis," though it could just as easily be called "staffarrhea." If you suspect this problem, what can you do next to verify the problem and apply solutions?

First, as in medicine, apply the lab tests. In this case there are several options:

- Exit interviews with departing staff to get candid feedback on their real feelings about your workplace.
- Handing out a simple written staff survey. Ask your staff on a 1 to 10 scale to rate the level of overall morale in the practice and what they would do to improve morale.
- Frequent one-on-one or small group meetings with the office manager or managing partner, which can be helpful to ferret out why you're losing staff.

- Conducting a community salary survey to see if you're underpaying compared to the local market rates.
- Pulling together all staff, or at least the staff in one department, for a group discussion on what the issues might be.

As for effective treatment regimens for teamitis, use what you learn during your survey work. The most common concern we hear from staffers is not related to hours or wages, but to doctor interaction with staff. Gentle physicians who stay close to and treat staff respectfully can get by with much lower wage rates than "Dr. Razor Wire."

We Are Behind in Our Patient Accounts Work. Collections Are Down. What's Up?

"Collectionopathy" may be the culprit. There are many potential root causes, so you need to examine several benchmarks:

- The time lag from your provision of a service to submission of a claim should be no more than 48 hours. The gold standard is to submit claims within 24 hours or less.
- In the typical general/geriatric practice, you should have no more than 12% of total open accounts out over 90 days. The tightest practices routinely achieve 8% or less.
- Maybe the problem is that you are understaffed. There are at least two ways to measure this. Divide the total annual collections of the practice by the number of all billing staff FTEs. The resulting figure should lie between \$800,000 and \$1.2 million in the typical practice. Another way to measure billing staff efficiency is to add all of the billing staff payroll hours in a year and divide this by the sum of all patient visits (including postoperative visits by convention) and all surgical cases. The resulting figure should be ±0.3 payroll hours per patient transaction.

If your practice's figures are materially different from these normative benchmarks, various treatment approaches may be in order:

- Any practice with more than one billing clerk should have someone who leads the billing department.
- If you don't have one already, create a detailed operations manual for your billing department.
- If you appear to have too few billing staff, based on the benchmarks above, it may be time to staff up to normal levels.
- If you appear to have excessive staff, consider trimming the ranks or redeploying staff to other areas of the practice.
- You should have at least two key operators (super users) for your practice management computer system; training on your system should be continuous.
- Ideally, the administrator (and in small and medium-sized practices, the managing partner) knows enough about patient accounts and your computer system that they can effectively post a charge, submit a claim, or review the status of an open account.

Each Year We Seem to Have Fewer and Fewer New Patients. What's Happening?

Perhaps your practice suffers from "promotional atrophy." To get a handle on this, take the following steps:

- Evaluate the local competition. Are they more visible than your practice? If so, is it because they're spending more marketing and advertising dollars or just spending more wisely?
- Examine your annual marketing budget. For general ophthalmology practices, it's typical and healthy to spend 2% to 5% of collections on marketing. For a refractive surgery practice, promotional outlays of 10% or higher are commonly required.
- Look at how you apportion your budget. Have you slivered the budget and spread your dollars too thinly to be effective in any one area? Are your dollars apportioned roughly pro rata to the natural sources of patients in your area?
- Do you jump from one promotional tactic to the next, never giving any execution enough time to build impressions?
- Is your marketing consistent? Do all of your ads look or sound like they came from the same branded company, or from several practices? The former is obviously preferred.
- Is the problem inside your practice? Remember: Nothing will make a flawed product fail faster than great marketing.
- Is someone in charge of and accountable for your marketing effectiveness?

Based on the results of this examination, you can then prescribe tactics to improve the number of new patients. These tactics may include increasing your budgetary commitments, firing an ineffective ad agency, diverting dollars to the tactics that work best in your area, or rebranding the entire practice to stand up to growing competition.

Our Schedule Is Booking Out Six Weeks. Our Doctors Are Running Ragged. Do We Need More Providers?

Let's call this one "hypomedicos." How do you know when you need another doctor? Again, turn to the lab reports:

- The typical, hardworking, full-time general ophthalmologist should be able to see 550 or more patient visits per month, perhaps 80% to 90% of this if practicing in one of the subspecialties. If the doctor is seeing fewer patients than this, determine the cause. Is it too few patients to see, too much socializing, or ineffective techs (leaving the doctors to repeat the history and early exam steps)?

- Is the rate-limiting resource really the doctors? Your clinic may just need a couple of additional lanes or techs. You should be able to transit about one patient visit per exam room hour. (To calculate this, take the number of total patient visits in a year and divide this by the number of complete exam rooms times 2080 hours per year.) You can tell if you have too many techs by multiplying the number of tech FTEs times 2080 hours per year and dividing the resulting figure by the number of patient visits per year. Norms are 0.8 to 1.0 tech payroll hours per patient visit in general practices, but they can rise to 1.3 in retinal practices, and about 1.1 in LASIK practices.
- Designate an office manager or head tech to quietly observe each of the doctors for a half day, writing down every example of wasted time and motion.

If you are over or under these benchmarks, it's relatively easy to add or subtract resources or patient volumes so your practice has an appropriate balance between doctor capacity and clinical work volumes.

• • •

A doctor has to memorize thousands of physiologic norms in the course of his or her training—and also has to know how to pair these up with precise diagnostic and treatment pathways. Happily, to be a highly effective administrator or physician-leader, you need to memorize only about 50 business norms to stay on top of the health of your practice.

CHAPTER 48

How Surgeons Can Help Themselves by Helping Their Management Team Thrive

Investing in management means building communication systems, business processes, feedback, and routines that let you scale the business and team as efficiently as possible.
—Fred Wilson

A good teacher must be able to put himself in the place of those who find learning hard.
—Eliphas Levi

Manage others the way you would like to be managed.
—Brian Tracy

On the way to becoming an eye surgeon, most ophthalmologists put in a lot of time not just learning but also teaching, either as formal teaching assistants during their university years, or less formally as the smartest student in the class, who helped fellow students with difficult subjects.

Wohl C, Pinto JB. *UP: Taking Ophthalmic Administrators and Their Management Teams to the Next Level of Skill, Performance, and Career Satisfaction, Second Edition* (pp 249-251). © 2021 Taylor & Francis Group.

The best and most successful surgeons, who go on to be the owners of vibrant practices, embrace a continuing role as a generous teacher and mentor. They do this at several levels:

- As clinicians, helping their patients make important treatment decisions
- As supervising physicians, helping younger doctors in a group practice polish their craft
- As business leaders, helping their administrators and mid-level department managers improve their skills

As the administrator of your practice it is your responsibility to determine if you and your management team are thriving or not—and if not, to figure out what steps need to be taken to move from "We're barely making it" to "We've got this." Your doctor-leader may believe that your positive attitude and dedicated long hours tell the whole story, but that is often not the truth.

The following is a list of ways your doctor-leaders can help make this happen in your practice. There are numerous, conscious ways of being a better educator.

- **Be involved with all new staff hires and promotions ... and demotions.** If you're too busy to interview the finalists for head tech or lead receptionist, you have weak grounds for complaining when the manager selected doesn't rise to your standards. Go beyond a perfunctory "Hello" to a deep interview with any new management staff and senior staff who are moving up the ladder. And every time a manager fails, don't leave it to your administrator alone to conduct the demotion or exit interview. Join the discussion. It's a splendid opportunity to improve not only the company's collective skill at picking leaders, but your own skills as a business owner.
- **Set the right tone, establish your practice as a learning organization.** What does that mean? It means you take the time to answer staff questions patiently. You attend staff meetings and present topics that will help staff better help your patients. Encourage that protocols and policies are not just passed along orally but memorialized in writing and periodically reviewed for potential improvements and clarifications. Objectively, the average department manager or administrator in your practice should be spending about as much time on formal continuing education as you do about 3% to 5% of their professional time, or roughly 1 day per month. Readings, group discussion of focused management topics germane to the company's challenges, formal conferences, and workshops all apply.
- **Stay personally involved in training senior management staff.** There are numerous outlets for this, starting with your administrator. Your practice manager may be skilled at accounting or billing or marketing or human resources (HR). But he or she is probably underinformed about the nuances of the products and services your practice sells (even after coming up the ranks as a technician before becoming a manager). Help your administrator understand the most common eye diseases and their treatment. Collaborate to discover together the economic and clinical impact of one course of treatment vs another. Help your billing manager learn how to conduct more thorough chart audits. Help your tech supervisor make a training video when a new piece of equipment is purchased.

- **Be generous with continuing education funding.** This goes beyond sending senior staff to national meetings. Encourage your administrator to scan for local community college courses in bookkeeping, HR management, and facilities management. Set up a tuition subsidy program for promising managers who could be more valuable to you if they finished college or picked up an advanced degree. All managers should have individual or group subscriptions to publications relevant to their specialist areas. Consider setting aside shelf space and obliging each manager to buy (at the practice's expense) one germane book per month, read it, and report a pearl or two they learned at a manager's meeting—and then have the book go into the practice's reference library. This can go beyond printed books. Audio management, executive effectiveness, and similar courses can make good use of morning and evening commuting time and of trips between satellite offices if you have a hub-and-spoke practice.
- **Provide abundant encouragement whenever you catch senior staff leading their staff effectively.** As a surgeon you were probably trained in a "gotcha" environment, jumped on by professors every time you missed a step or made an error. As a result, you quite likely apply the same method to your administrator and middle managers: Silence when their work is done well and stern reproach whenever you discover small errors. The fastest way to improve management's morale (and frankly, the morale of all lay staff) is to praise early and often, pointing out even the smallest performance gains you notice.
- **Develop a deeper level of strategic intimacy with your management staff.** We often perform this exercise with physician clients and their managers sitting together around a conference table. We hand out pens and paper, and ask everyone to "write down a description of the practice 5 years from now." The all-too-common result is that managers and doctors write down very differing visions of where they see the practice heading in the future. Strategic planning is a board-level responsibility that should be pursued in collaboration with the practice administrator and mid-level managers (who can help ensure the feasibility of your operational goals).
- **Ask for feedback.** Ask each of your senior staff members at frequent intervals, "Is there anything I could be doing to be a better practice owner? To back you up? To support your role as a leader here?" And then, take their advice. Along the way, be humble—when a manager fails, ask yourself, "How much of their failure was my responsibility?"

CHAPTER 49

Perking Up Your Practice Tempo With Greater Operational Agility

How Doctor-Leaders Can Help Their Administrators

Jack be nimble, Jack be quick,
Jack jump over the candlestick.
—Mid-19th century nursery rhyme

Quickness is the essence of the war.
—Sun Tzu

When you get to the top of the mountain,
keep climbing.
—Zen proverb

As professional fees languish in the years ahead, the winning practices will be those that can extract the most value out of their increasingly costly resource base. What's needed is more patient throughput per exam room per hour. More phone calls answered and cleared in a day. More insurance claims filed per shift.

The standards are rising. Margins are getting squeezed. The acceptable work pace a decade ago, for doctors and staff alike, is now looking kind of pokey.

Wohl C, Pinto JB. *UP: Taking Ophthalmic Administrators and Their Management Teams to the Next Level of Skill, Performance, and Career Satisfaction, Second Edition* (pp 253-255).

Here are 12 ideas that you (and your doctors, too!) can use for a zippier practice:

1. **Realize that everyone else takes their signals from you and the doctors.** As leaders in your practice, foster a sense of urgency. This can be expressed in numerous ways. Don't stroll down the hallway, stride. Encourage brief, to-the-point responses from your people. Provide quick, unwavering answers to staff questions without waffling. Give people realistic deadlines and goals, but here and there, also hand out "push" goals that might be barely attainable but will help the most promising members of your team grow faster. Don't verge into frantic territory. Try your best to combine the serious serenity of your high school principal with the tempo of a triple espresso.
2. **Arrive at the office early and start in high gear.** How early? For doctors, at least 30 minutes before the first patient's appointment. This will be a challenge if you are not a morning person. But in our experience, sluggish practices are generally owned by sluggish doctors, who arrive 30 minutes (even 3 hours!) after their first patient has been worked up. Only after you are disciplined personally as the practice owner is it fair for you to ask all staff to arrive on time and move briskly.
3. **Time is money.** Help staff understand the value of time and create a culture that squeezes as much value as possible out of every hour. In the typical solo practice, it costs more than $300 per hour to keep the doors open. Multiply that figure times the number of doctors in your practice, and you'll see you need to convey the urgency of using every hour to good purpose. (This doesn't only apply to lay staff; that subspecialist you employ is costing you $10 per minute in lost profits for every pause to check email.)
4. **Don't let urgency crowd out the endless pursuit of perfection.** We've often observed that our clients will ramp up their patient volumes, but their average collections per patient visit fall because they don't take the time to order special testing or help borderline patients consider surgery more thoughtfully.
5. **Compress old, accustomed time frames.** When is the next available routine appointment in your template? How much staff time does it take to check in and register a patient? How long after a patient is seen by the doctor does it take to check the patient out and make a new appointment? Post and submit a claim? Dictate a consult letter? Make a list of routine work like this you believe can be accomplished in less time, and then start working from the top of the list to speed up operations. (After you finish the list, be sure to recheck periodically to ensure that staff remain in high-tempo mode.)
6. **As the saying goes, work expands to fill the available time.** If you are overstaffed (or underbusy as a practice), you and your people will be conditioned to move at a slow pace. You can improve this by decreasing staffing levels and/or increasing patient volumes. And you don't need to make any permanent changes to prove just how effective these two moves might be. If you suspect you have one excess front desk clerk, sideline your weakest receptionist for a month (on a special project), and observe whether that person is really nonessential.

7. **Enforce personal responsibility.** Businesses don't get things done, people do. When you give a specific task to two people (or worse, the assembled staff at a practice meeting), then nobody is responsible. Every important project should have an owner, deadline, and written progress notes so that the project owner can report formally on progress and deadlines are less likely to drift.
8. **Consistency is a friend of speed.** If every tech informally develops a personal idiosyncratic way of working up patients, it is guaranteed that all but one tech (or maybe none) are preparing patients for the doctors in the best, fastest way. As a supervising physician or managing partner, work with your management team to encourage staff to write down the one, agreed-upon, best way to do everything. Then personally observe staff as they go through their paces: Are they following the accepted approach or drifting into old habits?
9. **Remember the old maxim, "Everything that can be measured can be improved."** Whether you are measuring big things (eg, project deadlines, annual profit margins) or small things (eg, work-up times, refracting accuracy), develop agreed-upon standards and targets.
10. **Be on the lookout for low-value activity.** You may have casually asked a staffer years ago to track visits per day or per week, data that have no practical value except on a spot-checking basis. Ask your people often, "Is there any part of your job that represents wasted time or busywork or an outdated approach that we should eliminate? How much time would this free up, and how would you use that time to better help our patients?"
11. **Replace poorly functioning work tools: Slow computers, outdated software, creaky photocopiers or testing equipment on their last legs.** Saving a few hundred dollars on delayed replacements can cost thousands in staff inefficiency and reduced job satisfaction.
12. **Becoming faster can be uncomfortable.** You, if you are incentivized for production goals, and your doctor business owners (and your patients, too) will obviously be rewarded by a brisk pace. How about staff? Not so much. They will need to work harder, and more intensely and intentionally. So, you need to be sure to reward gains in operational agility. If your efforts allow care for more patients with the same number of staff, consider a one-time discretionary bonus, selective raises, or a modest adjustment in wages across the board.

• • •

Of course, to be operationally nimble you also need to be strategically nimble. The majority of large practice boards and nearly all smaller-scale practice owners operate their organizations with no formal strategic grounding. Strategy and tactics are often confused. Strategic goals, like "grow our practice by 10% per year in net collections," need the support of tactical objectives such as "ramp up outreach and general consumer advertising to add 100 incremental new patients per month and outfit three more lanes." If you can combine strategic nimbleness with operational agility, your practice will be unstoppable.

CHAPTER 50

How to Seamlessly Add a New Associate Doctor to Your Practice

Anything you can do to stay organized and free up the creative side of your brain is a good thing.
—Chuck Hogan

Even if you are on the right track, you'll get run over if you just sit there.
—Will Rogers

No matter how many times you have expanded your professional staffing, it's an exciting time and a big deal when a new doctor joins your practice. But it's also an exhausting and detail-packed time. Your practice is composed of thousands of moving parts that can gum up quickly without a well-constructed onboarding plan.

The paperwork part can be simple if you prepare a checklist and assign one person to own responsibility for ensuring all items are completed by agreed-upon deadlines. Here is an incomplete summary of the highlights you have to nail:

Wohl C, Pinto JB. *UP: Taking Ophthalmic Administrators and Their Management Teams to the Next Level of Skill, Performance, and Career Satisfaction, Second Edition* (pp 257-261).

1. Employment contract (approved by your legal counsel and signed by the new doctor)
2. Background check (specific to your state permitted requirements), including Medicare exclusion screen
3. Relocation assistance as needed
4. All appropriate licenses and credentials confirmed
5. Professional liability insurance obtained
6. Credentialing at local hospitals, ambulatory surgical centers (ASCs), and with health insurance payers
7. Office signage, business stationery, website, and marketing materials updates
8. Orientation and communication about the practice's standards, care pathways, etc.
9. Introductions in the community; jump starting a formal outreach program
10. Advance appointment template preparation so the new doctor is busy, and cash is flowing as quickly as possible

Here is a sample document you can use to turn your checklist into a more detailed accountability document so you can avoid surprises, gaps, or missteps. Again, this list will likely be much longer and more granular in your setting:

New Doctor Onboarding Checklist

Task	Assigned To	Deadline	Completion Date	Progress Notes
Complete background checks, exclusion screens, licenses				
Employment contract signed				
Staff announcement regarding start date and onboarding plan developed				
Secure professional liability insurance				
Credentialing process for all payers/hospitals/ASCs (Be detailed—by payer and organization—on your list)				
Prepare onboarding plans and orientation kit (employee manual, staff contact list, prior internal newsletters, new hire forms, helpful how-to documentation)				

(continued)

New Doctor Onboarding Checklist (continued)

Task	Assigned To	Deadline	Completion Date	Progress Notes
Prepare orientation schedule, including meetings with all managers and assigned doctors to shadow				
Bio development and photo for website/marketing/announcements				
Update letterhead				
Order business cards				
Add to staff roster				
Assign office space, phone extension, etc.				
Patient appointment templates designed and opened				
Determine staffing needs based on anticipated patient volume				
Determine equipment and lane needs, if not already completed during the hiring process				
Order dictation equipment or add to dictation service/prepare for transcription service needed				
Order new signage for all offices				
IT prep (usernames/passcodes to all systems, add to appointment and billing systems)				
Schedule and complete electronic health record (EHR) training				
Keys for offices/security system codes				
Order white coats/scrubs with embroidered name				

Turning now to the first weeks of onboarding your new associate, recognize that first impressions still count. Even though your new doctor has visited the practice (hopefully more than once), it is another opportunity for positive impressions, and it is where opportunities to retain your new associate begin—only about 50% of partner-track eye surgeons ever actually make it to partner. We hear too often that new associates are dismayed at the tepid welcome they receive, which makes them wonder if they have made an error in practice choice. By the time the contract is signed and the new doctor arrives, your practice has made an expensive commitment. You want to make this hire stick.

The best onboarding and orientation schedule starts with an empty patient appointment template for the first week or longer (depending on the size of your practice and what there is to learn). This is not only smart, but also humane for the new doctor who wants to make excellent first impressions with each patient and the practice staff. Assign an experienced doctor in your practice as primary mentor for the associate's first year on staff. As the new doctor initially shadows a couple of doctors during clinic hours, practice goals and expectations about patient flow, customer service, staff support, and billing practices will be established and developed.

Another great onboarding exercise is to have each department manager spend an hour explaining what is accomplished in that department and by whom. This is an excellent opportunity for the manager to review the primary ways to be supportive to the new doctor. It's also a good time to for them to discuss what they will reasonably expect from one another. The new associate should review the practice operations manual, which every practice large enough to take on a second or subsequent associate should have on the shelf.

Another important tool, especially in larger settings, is an organizational chart showing the names and contact information for the new doctor to keep on hand. This facilitates a quick answer to the expected multitude of questions and can reduce new associate stress. It also takes a burden off you and your clinic manager, who will otherwise end up with all the questions, distracting in potentially unnecessary time-consuming ways.

For every new doctor, joining a new practice and a new community is not just a new career stage, but a life change. It can be a bit stressful and lonely. A proper social welcome is important. When we ask departing associates why they are leaving for a new practice, their common answer is, "Because this practice simply was not very welcoming … I didn't feel wanted here." Success factors include:

- A formal partner-level boss to report to and look to for support. A beer after work or a game of golf can work wonders to help young doctors feel a part of the team.
- Involvement as a frequent guest in the board room.
- All-provider dinners at least every quarter to discuss medicine and business and to develop social ties.
- Purely social gatherings of providers and their significant others a couple of times a year.

Even after several weeks in the practice, new associates will continue to raise questions about practice-specific policies, such as:

- EHR/e-prescribing/Merit-based Incentive Payment System expectations
- Billing, coding, and collections and auditing practices
- Patient and testing services flow
- Who the important inbound and outbound referral parties are and how they should be approached

In very large settings, where many new provider hires are made in a year, writing down a dynamic frequently asked questions cheat-sheet that is refined and added to over time can ensure that nothing is missed.

Be careful not to fall into the outdated perspectives the most senior doctors in your practice may have, viewing the onboarding process more casually, and saying, "I learned the hard way on my own and so can the new associate." In today's fast-paced environment, patient expectations are high from the outset. Documentation requirements are more demanding. Younger generation staff (and patients) are less forgiving.

In past generations, there were at least two new graduates for every available job. Today there are more than two jobs for every graduate, so you face a lot of recruitment competition, not just for this hire, but for every physician hire you will be making the rest of your career.

CHAPTER 51

Helping New Physician-Owners Become Better Practice Partners

Some people dream of success, while other people get up every morning and make it happen.
—Wayne Huizenga

To be successful, you have to have your heart in your business, and your business in your heart.
—Thomas Watson Sr.

Partners—compared to associate physicians—must take their business very seriously. Because partners have skin in the game, they need to know how the inner business game of ophthalmology works.

We are being asked more often by clients to coach their new partners on how to be better owners. Giving young doctors a jump start in this area not only makes them more self-assured, but also accelerates the pace at which they help you, as administrator, build a financially robust practice.

Business education for young partners is doubly important in multi-generational practices where young and old doctors don't yet mesh. In such practices, each generation has its own perspective on what makes a business succeed, and each doctor is simultaneously trying to build an individual practice.

Wohl C, Pinto JB. *UP: Taking Ophthalmic Administrators and Their Management Teams to the Next Level of Skill, Performance, and Career Satisfaction, Second Edition* (pp 263-266). © 2021 Taylor & Francis Group.

Even in practices where these conflicts don't exist overtly, the lack of business experience, along with natural differences in risk tolerance between young and old, can make boardroom meetings less productive and delay decision making.

As administrator, one way to help expedite a new partner's development as a more productive board member is to teach him or her general practice management concepts. This knowledge fosters a better understanding of the inner workings of your practice and how decisions impact others. It provides the informal education needed to understand why you take the steps you do to solve problems, and how and why you (and the board) utilize the information you collected to make decisions that help your practice become stronger and successful. Depending on your styles, this can be accomplished while sharing a weekly 15-minute coffee break or a 1-hour monthly scheduled education session. Taken together, the 10 topical areas that follow constitute a syllabus you can dive into one at a time.

These coaching points will help your newer partners jump start their understanding of how your practice functions business-wise and how they can contribute to your efforts to lead the practice forward.

1. **Financial and volumetric benchmarking.** One key to being a competent owner is to have the same command of the financial benchmarks for your practice as you do for your patients. Understanding financial reporting in your business is similar to knowing how to interpret your patients' exam data; substitute return on investment (ROI) for intraocular pressure (IOP) and you get the idea. By knowing the normal limits of either value, you are a better owner or a better doctor. Fortunately, there are only a few dozen norms to grasp, including things like tech payroll hours per visit, profit margin, and the cost of optical goods sold. With benchmarks like these, you can make data-driven decisions.
2. **Acting like a shareholder.** Adopt the decorum and behavior expected of an owner with higher responsibilities. As a business owner your fiduciary responsibility is to make decisions that are best for the overall practice, not for yourself alone. Ideally, you started thinking and acting this way from the beginning as an associate. You need to earn respect to be valued as a leader. As you graduate from associate to shareholder, your actions are viewed under an even higher-powered microscope by staff and peers.
3. **Teamwork.** The most fortunate doctors learned teamwork playing team sports in school. But if you didn't play sports (or played solo sports like tennis or golf), the most difficult part of becoming a partner may be learning good leadership, as well as good followership. This is leveraged if you are working in an especially large practice where teamwork has complexities and subtleties not present in smaller organizations.

4. **Problem solving.** Doctors don't need an MBA to become excellent business problem solvers. Think like a doctor, as you have already been trained, and use these skills to solve business problems. Review the subjective and objective data of the presenting problem, diagnose, apply treatment, reevaluate to see if the problem has cleared up, and, if not, apply another treatment. Repeat until solved.
5. **Communication.** There are important differences between how you communicate as a doctor and how you communicate as a member of a business team. In the room with a patient, while you may be collaborative to a degree, you are mostly directive. In a business setting, the emphasis is on collaboration (even if you think you have the one, right answer at the outset). One new role for young owners is to be part of (and sometimes lead) efficient, productive meetings. In working with young doctors, we often start here, because all the textbook knowledge in the world about how business works will not be useful if you can't effectively communicate.
6. **Human resource management.** Human resource management includes how to hire, fire, enforce policies consistently, follow employment law, and compose written performance standards. Even if this area is mostly handled by your management team, you need a sensitivity to applying fair policies consistently to all employees.
7. **Harnessing the power of owner-administrator collaboration.** The strongest practices are led by the dyadic pairing of a managing partner and an administrator. Even if it will be many years before a young doctor graduates to the managing partner position, it helps to learn early on how this common management structure works (and how variations on doctor-administrator collaboration often lead to practice failure).
8. **Understanding the role of mid-level management.** Mid-level managers have titles like optical manager, director of technical services, and billing coordinator. These positions boost the core strength of your practice. Mid-level managers have a challenging role. They are often working side-by-side with their team as working supervisors. One minute they are leaders, the next minute they are a follower to upper-level management or doctors. Understanding their specific responsibilities and common challenges will help you understand the depth of their role and how you can help them develop as leaders in their own right.
9. **Developmental stages.** Children growing up pass through developmental stages that all vigilant parents observe. Practices also have developmental stages, based on their scale rather than age. For example, a solo practitioner and her staff can function smoothly with less formal written communication as compared to larger practices. In larger practices, in order to eliminate inefficiencies and staff confusion, it becomes necessary to develop care pathway policies and procedures that apply to all technicians and doctors. Young doctors need to become as sensitive as young parents to these natural stages of practice development, and work with management to recognize developmental lags.

10. **Marketing and practice development.** The average practice grows at about 5% in visits and revenue dollars per year. Below this figure, you are likely losing market share and creating an environment where the doctors start to compete with each other for limited numbers of patients. Large practices have formal marketing managers. But in the average practice with just two to three providers, everyone owns the marketing function. Doctors need to learn effective outreach discipline and customer service. Clerks need to stay on top of recall. The administrator is often on the front line, placing ads. Young owners need to find their own way to contribute to practice growth.

• • •

Becoming an effective partner and board member can sometimes feel as difficult as becoming an excellent surgeon. It doesn't happen overnight or magically. It takes a foundation of basic concepts combined with an interest in business affairs, close observation, patience, ambition, and ongoing mentoring. The business of medicine has nearly as much intellectual content as medicine itself and is a fascinating next course of study for young surgeons. Collaborating early in your career with your administrator and fellow business partners will catapult your business education.

Note to administrators: Although this chapter is intended to help new partners become better owners faster, the same concepts may be applied to any of your older owners who may have failed to develop in this critical area.

Quick-Start Quiz

Many of our readers are familiar with Pinto's Ten Commandments for Surgeons, which have become a classic in the profession. How many of these are you following?

Pinto's Ten Commandments for Surgeons

1. Hire the best people you can afford. Treat them right.
2. Provide staff with 1 hour of education for every 79 hours of work.
3. Keep tomorrow's appointment book 100% full.
4. Treat every patient as though they were your only customer.
5. Ask every patient to refer a friend.
6. Know your numbers. Cold.
7. Find a surgeon more competent than you and copy what they do.
8. Sweat every detail. Even the ones that bore you.
9. Financial success is measured in profit per hour not cases per month.
10. Live on less than 80% of your after-tax income. Invest the rest intelligently.

CHAPTER 52

Benefits of the Physician–Administrator Dyadic Leadership Model

The "dyad" is a partnership where an administrative leader is paired with a physician leader. An effective dyad is frequently referred to as a "work marriage"—the two partners balance each other's skills and weaknesses and work as a cohesive team toward a common goal.

—The Advisory Board Company

A majority of ophthalmic practices today pursue in reality—if not in name—a so-called *dyadic leadership model*. This model has the following chief features, whether the practice is small or large, and whether the practice has intentionally set up a dyadic approach by design or has organically arrived at this model inadvertently:

- A physician-owner is nominated, with a greater or lesser degree of formality, as the managing partner, president, or chairman of the practice.
- This physician works closely with the administrator. Each has written, board-approved roles, and they stay in their own lanes.

Wohl C, Pinto JB. *UP: Taking Ophthalmic Administrators and Their Management Teams to the Next Level of Skill, Performance, and Career Satisfaction, Second Edition* (pp 267-272).

- Both halves of the dyad work as hard on their relationship as they do on the practice, with frequent meetings and discussions that are deep enough to affirm that both parties are mostly on the same page, while respecting small differences.
- A successful co-managing relationship between the doctor-leader and lay administrator has much in common with effective parenting:
  - Shared values and standards
  - Shared vision for future priorities
  - Speaking publicly with a single voice
  - Consistency and reliability and predictable follow-through
  - No disagreements in front of the "children"
  - Seen as a unified force commanding respect
  - Not allowing the "children" to play "mom" against "dad"

As effective as this approach to practice leadership is, many practices have still not jumped on the dyadic bandwagon. Or, they are incompletely on board with the concept.

We often see the results of this in client practices. In some settings, even some larger practices, there is no managing partner, and the administrator is obliged to run a circuit from partner to partner to get things done.

In some settings, the physician and lay administrator are competitive rather than collaborative. They unduly poach responsibilities and authorities from each other's territories.

In other settings, we don't see outright conflict, but rather a relinquishment of responsibility; the managing partner who is more figurehead than leader and the administrator who has given up managing, saying, "What's the point? My doctor is going to want to do it his way, anyway."

Here are seven ideas to help you improve an existing dyadic leadership structure, or to establish a high-functioning dyadic leadership model where none presently exists.

1. The doctor-leader should be formally authorized by the board to lead. The managing partner position should have a written job description (see example later in this chapter) and a small honorarium (in the range of $1500 to $5000 per month, depending on the size of the practice). There should be a formal vote for the managing partner, and a term of 2 years with no term limits is best (a talented individual can be voted in for successive terms). A shorter term makes the new managing partner an immediate lame duck with little authority. Don't make the mistake of having every partner take a turn at being managing partner, run this critical aspect of your company as a meritocracy. The managing partner's performance should be reviewed formally by the board annually, or more often in the event of poor performance. Managing partners should be subject to mid-term removal.
2. Physician-leaders need to put in the time. In the average ±$5 million private practice, it's typical for the managing partner to spend about 8 hours per week at the job. Most new managing partners fear this will steal time from their work as an ophthalmologist and result in a pay cut, but this fear is unfounded. Empirically, we have seen managing partners only increase their income by being more engaged with the details of the practice and finding ways to increase the efficiency of their clinical life.

3. Administrators need to be comfortable sharing information and power. At the outset of launching a dyadic leadership model, and perhaps voting in a first-time managing partner, there can be a multimonth settling-in period. The new managing partner can be overgrasping and starting to take on some of the administrator's authorities. The administrator can understandably, almost unconsciously, withhold information from the managing partner in an effort to retain control. Any emerging conflict within the dyad that can't be reduced directly by the physician–administrator pair needs to be addressed by the board. In a few cases, a new administrator or a different managing partner is indicated.
4. Because the underlying relationship and trust between the administrator and managing partner is so critical, wise boards take administrator sentiments into consideration when selecting a new managing partner. Although the administrator may not have a formal vote in the boardroom, it's best to hear the administrator's views on which board member they could work with most effectively.
5. There has to be a good temperamental fit between the physician-leader and the administrator. They have to like and respect each other's expertise and role. In ideal settings, the administrator learns just as much about medicine and surgery as the managing partner learns about business.
6. There has to be a written strategic plan. Whether you are a doctor-leader or an administrator, it's hard to lead or manage effectively if the company does not have a board-approved business plan. This plan, which can be as short and informal as a few pages in less challenging or less ambitious settings, should discuss the 3- to 10-year intended future of the company, and nominate the desired growth rate, service area, service mix, provider mix, relations with other market participants, and succession details. The plan should be updated annually.
7. The managing partner needs to be a member of the practice's management committee. What's a management committee? In most settings this group, led by the administrator, includes the managing partner, the administrator, and all of the department heads (eg, technical services, billing, reception/call center/records, optical, ambulatory surgical center director). In the strongest practices, this group meets biweekly and is chiefly responsible for collaborating to ensure that operations are polished and projects are completed.

• • •

An effective dyadic partnership between doctor and administrator does not arise overnight. As our colleague, consultant Craig Piso, PhD, puts it, "Dyadic leadership is excruciatingly simple and intuitive in principle. But it is sometimes subtle and frustratingly slow to emerge when applied in your own practice, even with the best intent." You'll know you're getting better at it when the following signs emerge in your own practice:

- The board and entire staff view the managing partner and practice administrator as a single unit speaking with one voice.
- Members of the practice come to trust the benevolent intent of their leaders, who are acting on behalf of the entire group.
- There is growing respect for the written values, rules, and structure that the dyad represents and is entrusted to secure.

- The practice team is not just grudgingly acquiescent to the dyad's role and authority but is periodically inspired by its vision as well.
- Such practices and their constituent staff members will often start taking bigger risks, because their core is strong enough to withstand any misjudgment or lapses in execution.

Sample Managing Partner Position Description

Reports to: Board of Directors
Term of office: 2 years with no term limits
Compensation: $1850 per month
Core skills and resources inventory:

- Five to 10 hours per week for internal/external meetings and data analysis
- Financial acumen sufficient to evaluate monthly reports and to monitor progress toward agreed-upon volume and profit targets
- The ability (and widely held credibility) to actively mentor fellow doctors and to not avoid uncomfortable situations or conflicts
- The ability to communicate directly and clearly, in writing and verbally
- Sufficient discipline to stick to board-agreed directives and not succumb to "mission drift"

Core duties:

- **Broad charter.** To work with the practice's administrator to help turn the board-mandated mission, goals, and policies into daily operations.
- **Budget and performance forecasting.** Oversight, with administrator and external practice accounting resources, over the preparation of monthly financial statements and volume performance summary reports. Participates in the preparation of a forward-looking pro forma forecast of anticipated practice performance. Is the doctor's disciplinarian, responsible for ensuring that an appropriate cost-benefit analysis is conducted for all new projects, policies, capital equipment purchases, and other initiatives.
- **Profitability review and enhancement.** Works with administrator to coach doctors on where they stand compared to their profit and volume goals; intervenes briskly if by-doctor volumes or revenues lag.
- **Committee positions.** Member of the practice management committee composed of selected senior staff, which manages day-to-day operations; chair of the practice's board of directors.
- **Outreach and ongoing market assessment.** Helps to maintain ongoing, senior-level contacts with the practice's sources of patients and with payers in the regions.
- **Planning and development.** Works with administrator to prepare and at least annually revise the practice's strategic and business operations plan; leads the board approval process for each subsequent edition.

- **Recruitment.** Involved in provider and senior staff recruitment activities.
- **Practice project and action monitoring.** Provides board oversight for the continued maintenance of a comprehensive action grid summarizing all key practice activities and projects, those responsible for their completion and agreed-upon deadlines; in consultation with shareholder doctors has authority to reward and reprimand the practice's lay managers for their performance in meeting agreed-upon goals and objectives.
- **Spending authority.** Holds, with the administrator, complete on-budget spending authority; subject to review and oversight, has off-budget discretionary spending authority up to the limit of $5000 total impact before consulting with shareholder doctors. This spending authority may be subject to ongoing adjustment based on practice performance.
- **Clinical practices oversight and provider discipline.** Uses internal providers and outside advisory resources to conduct risk management, utilization, and quality assurance reviews; in consultation with the board has the ability to suspend or revise any clinical practices believed to be inappropriate. Is responsible for applying a progressive discipline system to misbehaving partner and associate doctors, ranging from informal peer counseling to termination (the latter with board oversight).
- **Conflict resolution.** Works to resolve provider-to-provider conflicts, including optometric scope-of-practice issues, patient assignment, and issues of which doctors should be providing which clinical and surgical services.

Managing Partner's Ten-Point Monthly Checklist

1. At least two formal monthly meetings with the practice administrator and review of monthly reporting, accountability/action grid (updated biweekly), graphs, and financial forecasts
2. A rereading of the practice's strategic plan and asking yourself: "Are we still sticking to the plan?"
3. Attendance and participation at the regular senior managers' meetings
4. Prepare for and conduct an owners' monthly board meeting
5. Review of and action regarding any open provider discipline matters
6. Minimum of 2 hours per month (in aggregate, just a few minutes a day) spent walking the halls, visiting informally with support staff, asking questions and praising performance
7. A mental scan of all external relationships (eg, hospitals, referral sources, competitors, payers, vendors), follow-up written, phone, or face-to-face action as needed
8. A lunch, breakfast, or similar meeting with one practice department head per month and with one of the practice's doctors (separate or combined meeting as desired)

9. Reading/scanning of one general management book per month and reading/scanning of a business weekly or monthly such as *Business Week* or *The Economist*; share relevant articles with the management staff and board members
10. Monthly exercise; ask yourself, "What have I done this month to improve my weakest management skill, be it gathering information, making decisions, or taking action?"

CHAPTER 53

For Doctors

On Choosing and Managing the Right Practice Administrator

The best executive is the one who has sense enough to pick good men to do what he wants done, and self-restraint to keep from meddling with them while they do it.
—Theodore Roosevelt

I am convinced that nothing we do is more important than hiring and developing people. At the end of the day you bet on people, not on strategies.
—Lawrence Bossidy

Great vision without great people is irrelevant.
—Jim Collins

Great practices are built from the top down. After choosing where you want to practice and the right colleagues to practice with, the most important enterprise decision you have as a private practice owner or institutional department chair is which lay leader will manage your business.

Lay practice leaders come in five basic flavors:

1. The chief of staff, who is little more than an executive assistant to a physician-owner-operator. Such individuals may receive a salary ranging up to $75,000 and may have the title "manager," but their authority is sharply limited. Everyone really reports to the doctor-boss.

Wohl C, Pinto JB. *UP: Taking Ophthalmic Administrators and Their Management Teams to the Next Level of Skill, Performance, and Career Satisfaction, Second Edition* (pp 273-278).

2. The office manager, who, despite the low-octane title, may have full-charge responsibility for a small boutique practice. The office manager is typically charged with day-to-day operations but has no material spending or hire-and-fire authority. Depending on the manager's experience and the market, office managers have a base salary today ranging from $60,000 to about $80,000.
3. The administrator, is a kind of "CEO-lite," responsible for both operations and profitability, but in most cases with relatively limited off-budget spending authority. The vast majority of ophthalmic practices in the United States today, being in the $2- to $5-million bandwidth, employ an administrator. What does that cost them? In the rural United States, the administrator of a large practice may earn less than the office manager of an urban practice, but the wide-ranging base salary for experienced administrators today is $60,000 to $150,000.
4. The executive director, who typically leads practices with revenue in the range of $5 million to $20 million, is predictably hard-charging and career-focused. In alignment with the managing partner this leader takes command of the practice boardroom ... and is often granted a much higher level of discretionary spending than more junior administrative colleagues. Executive directors pull in $150,000 to $200,000 as a base wage, not because the title is more impressive than an administrator's, but because executive directors have higher skill sets and personal commitment. A $10-million practice needs four times the leader of a $5-million practice.
5. The CEO is generally found in only the largest practices. He or she is granted significant executive and financial authority over the practice. CEOs cue up long-term strategies and budgets for final board approval, and, if they are the right person in the right job, their board need only provide light-handed oversight, not fiat control. The highest-paid ophthalmic executives today enjoy physician-level base salaries ranging to $300,000 and perquisites taking this figure much higher.

As you can see from this, no matter if you have a small or large practice, you are going to spend about 1% to 5% of cash flow to hire and support the brains of the outfit.

With that kind of money at stake, you want to find the right kind of leader-manager, someone suited to the scale and aspirations of your practice. It's as big an error to undershoot and select a junior executive assistant to run a large practice as it is to overshoot and hire a CEO for a small-time operation.

Here are some considerations to help you get it right the first time around.

- The hardest practice to manage is the mid-sized practice. You need to know how to do every job in the practice and have a balanced portfolio of leadership and management skills. Small, solo practices have fewer moving parts and are relatively easy to manage. Enormous practices, captained by CEOs and executive directors, have a deep bench of middle managers with lots of redundant in-house skills, and they are comparatively easy to manage (even if very difficult to lead).
- Decide whether you need more of a leader, more of a manager, or a blend of the two. Leadership and management are overlapping but very different skills. This is frustratingly evident in the functioning of most elected officials. The leadership chops needed to stand up and charismatically frame up a mission and pull people along in that direction has little correlation to getting the job done. In personnel

management circles, a great leader who speaks well but can't perform is called a communicative incompetent. Don't hire one of these.

- No administrator has a complete skill set. Some are excellent at personnel issues but weak at finance. Some are weak at marketing but a whiz at operating efficiencies. Know your prospective administrator's core competencies before you make the hire and realize that any missing skills will either need to be learned, supplied by someone else in the practice, or outsourced.
- The core competencies of the administrator you hire should coincide with your practice's greatest current and anticipated needs. If you're financially on the ropes, you need numeracy. If referral source outreach is flagging, you need selling skills. If customer service is your weakest link, make sure your new hire has a proven record of improving service performance in a similar setting.
- Practice management and leadership is only partially a so-called *learned profession*. Unlike law, engineering, or medicine, there is no agreed-upon or required standard of licensure, no test to pass. An advanced business degree provides an excellent academic education, but unfortunately, we've seen more MBAs blow up practices than up-through-the-ranks managers with associate degrees. Look for the right mix of education and experience.
- Hiring a high-energy, eager person to lead your practice is necessary, but insufficient. To increase the odds of business success, one needs to hire gung-ho people who have a proven track record of analogous performance in analogous settings. Hiring an ex-hospital administrator for your very large practice may sound logical, but the skill set needed to run a 400-bed hospital is profoundly different than the skills needed to run even the largest ophthalmology practice.
- Executives who are enthusiastic but inexperienced, when paired with a high-demand boss who labels all requests "RED HOT" will collect more open, incomplete projects than closed accomplishments. If you are a high-demand practice owner, make sure you hire someone who can prioritize and stand up to your criticism about why last week's hot project hasn't been launched yet.
- Unless you are acting as the physician-administrator of your practice, and just need an executive assistant to carry out your ideas and orders, big brains are obligatory in your top executive. But intelligence is an incomplete substitute for raw time commitment.
- Beyond the time commitment of your administrator, the managing partner of the practice must commit time and attention to the company. Even the strongest CEO of the largest practices in the United States that we see firsthand struggle if their lead physician counterpart is time-poor or disengaged. In practical terms, this typically translates to the effective managing partner of a solo to five-owner practice spending up to 8 hours per week on leadership duties, and the managing partners of larger practices commonly putting in 12 hours or more per week.

- Management and leadership are contact sports. To be successful, and achieve the shortest cycle time between finding and fixing a problem, everyone who touches each problem has to be in the same room together. Ideally, in a group practice with numerous providers, the doctor's personal offices (or workstation pods in a modernized office space) are arrayed around a large board table, and the administrator's private office is in this same suite. An executive assistant, bookkeeper or CFO, and IT exec are nearby. This increases the odds of owners and managers running into each other throughout the day, developing stronger relationships, and applying better solutions to problems they find faster.

In addition to these already-numerous reasons we've discussed for why it is essential for you to place the utmost importance on finding and managing a stellar administrator or office manager, here is one more. Because nowhere, at least in the business sphere of your practice, is excess human churning costlier and more frustrating than with your practice's administrator, whose likely tenure in the average setting is about 6 years, more or less.

Based on our experience, about 40% of practice owners are ecstatic about their administrators or practice managers, another 50% or so are equivocal or worse, and 10% are currently on the hunt for a new lay leader or will be within the next year.

Lots of essentials go into assessing the fit of your current administrator, selecting a new practice leader if and when this becomes necessary, as well as upping the odds for long tenure. Here are seven elements to consider in your own setting.

1. **A desire to lead.** Those who work their way into leadership and are also competent at it are foremost people with a desire to lead. Of course, this trait alone, in the absence of aptitude, can backfire. A mere desire to lead does not always align with one's ability to do so. A desire to lead is a necessary but insufficient condition for holding down an administrative job. From John's face-to-face discussions with thousands of mid- and senior-level managers over the last 35 years in the field, it's clear that not all administrators are eager for the challenge. Many are in fact reluctant leaders, elevated above their innate comfort level and competency by well-meaning doctors. Seen from most surgeons' perspectives, this would be like taking on a cataract practice composed of nothing but complications. The exceptional surgeon might relish the challenge, but the average surgeon would dread coming to work. If your administrator is out of his or her depth and knows it, it will be both a miserable and disappointing experience on the job.
2. **Technical competence.** Put this in doctoring terms. If called upon, we could probably fake it and talk to a patient as though we knew what is happening to his or her eye and how we were going to treat it. But we've never mastered the body of technical skills to be able to competently do the job. Eventually, perhaps disastrously, we would be discovered. In the business sphere, the highest technical hurdle is economic analysis. Every effort should be made to ensure that the administrator is either already a master of the benchmarks, graphs, and statistics needed to competently assess your practice's health, or is at least progressing toward mastery in this area.

3. **Time commitment.** Semi-retired ophthalmic icon and pal, Dr. John Corboy, quips, "If you're not smarter than your competition, you had better work harder and longer than they do." Ophthalmology doesn't cleave to banker's hours. The typical practice administrator, at a minimum, must make a 45-hour-per-week commitment to the job. And 55 hours or more per week is not unusual, including conferences, industry readings, evening meetings, and the rest of it.
4. **Vigor.** The best and longest-tenured administrators we know tend to be fit and vigorous. This has nothing to do with age. I (John) fondly remember one large client's executive director, who well into his 60s would race me up three flights of stairs to his office. And win each time. Dealing with intense people-driven problems all day—and often into many late evenings—takes a level of energy and durability that only the most fortunate and competent administrators possess in abundance. It's a simple question: Does your current manager have the juice needed to lead your company?
5. **Face time with the practice's medical leader.** Your administrator will languish without regular face-to-face meeting time with the managing partner of your practice. This roughly weekly meeting should be arranged and kept as formally as a patient appointment time. In addition to one-on-one time, the best administrators, working as a collaborative duo with their managing partners will meet every 2 to 4 weeks with the mid-level managers of the practice (head tech, billing supervisor, etc). These management committee meetings are a time to hear first-hand how things are going in every corner of the company and sense the level of respect your administrator commands. And they provide a wonderful opportunity to send a signal to middle management that your administrator and his or her team enjoy the board's full support. (What? You say that your practice has not yet formally selected a managing partner? No matter what else you have on your plate for the rest of this year, that's job #1.)
6. **Very clear, written expectations about performance.** Sometimes, when I ask boards what they expect from their administrator this year, I get blank stares. What's worse, I get the same blank expression when I ask their administrator, "What does your board expect of you?" Every practice, even the smallest, should have a punch list of tactical goals for the year. An example would include large and small things like:
    - Complete Dr. Smith's buy-in transaction
    - Activate the new satellite office in Centerville
    - Launch a new vision screening program for older adults
    - Add two more techs
    - Boost practice profit margins from 32% to 36% by the end of the fiscal year
    - Refinish the reception chairs
    - Change over to the new phone system
    - Go live with electronic health records

    Your list should be reviewed at least monthly at a board level and will ideally show each task, the manager who owns it, the deadline, and a few updated progress notes.

7. **And, finally, there needs to be a sense of backing and support from the top.** This doesn't mean that you should avoid frank discussions about performance gaps. Unfortunately, ophthalmologists, like most professionally trained people, are natural-born critics. They are fast to criticize and slow to praise. If you want a good manager to grow with the practice and become a great manager, the dominant message has to be, "We admire you and appreciate your work for us and our staff and patients. We think of you as a professional peer, someone as competent and professional and striving at what you do as we as doctors are at what we do." Remember that in your position of power as a practice owner, with your administrator's fate and fortune in your hands, even an unearned stern glance can be demoralizing for weeks. To do the best job, your administrator needs to know he or she is liked, admired, appreciated, and secure.

• • •

Half of all ophthalmic practices in the United States perform below average, which means that if you are reading this, your business has 50-50 odds of being in trouble today. Improving this, and improving your practice's frank viability in the challenging years ahead, starts at the top with an above-average administrator.

CHAPTER 54

A Practice Management Pop Quiz for You and Your Administrator

Education's purpose is to replace an empty mind with an open one.
—Malcolm Forbes

Change is the end result of all true learning.
—Leo Buscaglia

After 25 years of formal education, the last thing you probably want to take right now is another pop quiz. But this one is different—and perhaps more directly predictive of your future economic success than any other you've been obliged to take. So bear with us.

Here are five questions. About half of all ophthalmic administrators in the United States, and a somewhat lower percentage of eye surgeons, can nail this test.

Right below the question set is an answer key. Let's be really lenient and call 60% a passing grade. But don't cheat and look at the answers until you've completed the quiz.

Wohl C, Pinto JB. *UP: Taking Ophthalmic Administrators and Their Management Teams to the Next Level of Skill, Performance, and Career Satisfaction, Second Edition* (pp 279-282).

1. A solo cataract surgery practice sees 500 patient visits per month, including postoperative visits. How many technicians (including working up patients, testing, and scribing) does this practice need to employ?
   a. 4.0
   b. 2.9
   c. 1.5
   d. None of the above
2. This same practice performs an average of 60 cataract surgeries per month. Which of these statements best describes the surgical density of this practice?
   a. About average. The typical eye surgeon seeing 500 visits per month is going to generate about 60 surgical cases per month.
   b. Very low. This must be a very hesitant surgeon.
   c. Quite good. This doctor has three times the surgical density of the average practice.
   d. Extremely high. This surgeon's surgical density suggests that he or she must be coercing patients into having unnecessary surgery.
3. A three-surgeon, general suburban practice with $3.8 million in annual collections spends $1.4 million each year on lay staffing (excluding OD, MD, and DO providers) and $300,000 on office facilities, including rent and utilities. Would you say this practice's staffing and facilities costs are:
   a. High
   b. Low
   c. Typical, right around where they should be
4. This same practice employs a total of 27 lay staff. Would you say these support staffers on average are:
   a. Overpaid
   b. Underpaid
5. A five-partner mixed subspecialty practice, including pediatrics and retinal care, has a 40% profit margin. All of the doctors are paid with a simple formula: They receive 40% of their individual collections. How would you characterize their financial arrangement?
   a. Just fine, no need to change
   b. Pretty close, but the board should hold back a slush fund of profits, as by paying everyone 35% of their collections, and then distributing the balance at the end of the year to the partners who are most deserving of a bonus
   c. Way off, the pediatric ophthalmologist is probably overpaid and the retinal surgeon is probably underpaid
   d. All of the above, depending on the sentiments of the owners

Answers

1. **b**—In the typical general practice, one needs about 1.0 technician payroll hours per patient visit. With 500 visits per month, that's about 500 hours of tech time monthly. There are 173 payroll hours (including vacation time and sick leave) in the average month for a single full-time-equivalent (FTE) worker. If we divide 500 hours of needed time by 173 hours per FTE, we get 2.9 FTEs, that's the number of techs a practice like this needs to employ, at least on paper. They may be able to get by on slightly less if all the techs are seasoned pros, and they may need more backup assistance if the practice sees a higher volume of pathology (with older, slower, sicker patients who need more testing and treatment).
2. **c**—The average ophthalmic practitioner in a general practice generates one cataract case (one operated eye) for every ±25 patient visits. This figure can be more than 40 visits per case in a young surgeon's practice and as low as five or fewer in a mature surgeon's office or in a practice that co-manages care with outside optometrists. In this case, we have a surgical density of 500 visits, divided by 60 cases, for a surgical density of 8.3 visits per case, which is about three times the average figure seen.
3. **a**—Staffing and facilities costs are both much higher than the normal range in this practice. Let's examine staffing costs first. The typical general practice spends 28% to 32% of cash flow on so-called fully burdened staffing—inclusive of wages, benefits, and taxes. This practice is spending $1.4 million on staffing, divided by $3.8 million in collections, or about 37%. If staffing costs were brought into line with norms (let's say 30% of collections), each of the three partners would receive a roughly $89,000 annual pay raise.

   Turning to facility costs, the normal range is to spend 4% to 6% of cash flow on office quarters. This practice is spending $300,000 divided into $3.8 million in collections, or 7.9% of cash flow on office space and utilities, much higher than normal for a suburban practice. (This higher percentage would be acceptable if the practice was in the center of an expensive city, or if it had just built a new facility a little larger than needed and was going to take a few years to grow into it.)
4. **a**—Dividing this practice's $1.4 million annual payroll by 27 staff means the average lay worker here is making almost $52,000 per year. That figure might have to be lived with in a market like Manhattan or San Francisco. But the average fully burdened cost per full-time staffer (averaging together everyone from file clerks to CEOs) in a suburban practice is closer to $45,000 per year. (It can be $35,000 in the rural United States.) So, staff in this practice are being overpaid by about 15%. This could be addressed in several ways, including:
   - By living with the problem and accepting the drag on profits
   - By reducing wages and/or benefits to market levels
   - By organizing the practice to generate more revenue and profit per patient visit, which won't bring down staffing costs, but will reduce costs as a percentage of cash flow
   - By reducing staff head count and trimming hours here and there (eg, sending staff home early on quiet days)

5. **d**—"All of the above" is the correct answer. There are hundreds of potential partner compensation models. These are influenced by numerous factors: the difficulty of recruiting subspecialist, practice cost structures, capitated managed care payments, and boardroom bullying. Even when you think you've devised the best possible formula, and everyone's happy, something changes to throw it off: a contract is lost, a high-producing surgeon joins the group, or a senior partner slows down. For this reason, a larger practice like this one should have a standing compensation committee of the board (ideally, composed of a high producer, a low producer, and the practice's CPA). This comp committee meets annually and presents its recommendation to the board to preserve or revise the current formula.

Add your correct answers. Did you hit 60% or higher? Study the answers you missed, and apply this same pop quiz to the real world of your own practice.

Appendices

APPENDIX A

Administrator Career Satisfaction Rank and Rate

Name: ____

Date: ____

Administrators' satisfaction with their professional situations is always multifactorial. Please read each item on the left and enter A/B/C and 1 to 10 scores to the right in the two rank and rate columns in the form following. Omit/ignore any items that don't apply to your situation.

When finished, review any high-level ("A" priority) items that have a lower satisfaction score. For each such item, write down a brief plan for how you might increase the 1 to 10 score this year.

Wohl C, Pinto JB. *UP: Taking Ophthalmic Administrators and Their Management Teams to the Next Level of Skill, Performance, and Career Satisfaction, Second Edition* (pp 285-288).

Variables Affecting an Administrator's Current Professional Satisfaction	Rank: How Important Is This to You? (A, B, or C) *A=High* *B=Medium* *C=Low*	Current Satisfaction Score (1 to 10) *1=Low* *10=High*
Compensation, including benefits, which is on balance equitable, proportionate to effort, and in line with market rates for administrator earnings		
The community where one lives and access to desired amenities: Scenery, culture, recreation, spouse's career opportunities, child education options, etc.		
Managing partner or solo owner: Professional harmony, the ability to speak the truth or make an unpopular recommendation for the benefit of the practice without fear or threat of job loss		
Board and associate doctor relationships: Professional harmony, the absence of major conflict, our ease of reaching reasonable compromise		
A respected, appropriate voice in practice-wide policy making		
Staff: Working relationships, competency, ability to make hire-and-fire recommendations that are reasonably followed		
Access to needed resources from practice owners: staff, facilities, technology, advertising/marketing promotion, etc.		

(continued)

Variables Affecting an Administrator's Current Professional Satisfaction	**Rank: How Important Is This to You? (A, B, or C)** *A=High* *B=Medium* *C=Low*	**Current Satisfaction Score (1 to 10)** *1=Low* *10=High*
Vendors: Reasonable authority and control over decisions that impact expenses and services for which I may be held accountable		
Independence: An administrator's ability to practice the profession without undue oversight or control from above (while always yielding to best practices and overall practice goals)		
Bonding and attachment to a cause greater than oneself: In most group practices, the collaborative delivery of superior eye care in a rapidly changing health care market provides feelings of pride, security, and solidarity		
Work/life balance: Not feeling chronically overwhelmed or burned out		
My greatest professional satisfaction this past year was __________________. It was recognized and appreciated.		
My greatest professional frustration this past year was __________________. It was recognized, and steps are being taken that will help me improve this situation.		

(continued)

Variables Affecting an Administrator's Current Professional Satisfaction	**Rank: How Important Is This to You? (A, B, or C)** *A=High* *B=Medium* *C=Low*	**Current Satisfaction Score (1 to 10)** *1=Low* *10=High*
The owners/board prepare written goals with me. At least annually, progress is evaluated and suggestions for improvement are made. I feel supported by the owner/board to improve my skills or knowledge.		
Written personal career goals are developed and revisited annually. I am free to reach for continuous professional growth.		
Other:		
Other:		

APPENDIX B

Doctors and Administrators

Actors on the Same Stage

Dear Doctor:

You asked me today how I was doing. I appreciated that, I really did. I told you, "Everything is great," and then we went our separate ways down the hall. You to clinic, me to my office.

Here's what your administrator—probably almost every administrator—is really thinking, even though she doesn't tell you.

You see, our jobs really aren't that different. We both gather information, make decisions, secure consent from our respective "patients," and do our best to treat problems at their root. Like you, when I'm walking through the clinic, I'm trying to solve four problems at the same time. My mind is racing between:

1. Why is the clinic flow delayed today?
2. How do we recruit that terrific candidate and stay within budget?
3. How would be best to teach Dr. Young to improve his documentation and coding?
4. What interesting spreadsheet can I create for the upcoming quarterly finance meeting?

On the way back to my office, I am approached by at least three people with their own issues. I listen, respond to their concerns, and continue on.

When you see me and I look like I'm at the end of my tether, don't be overly concerned. I probably have more capacity and will finish the week strong.

When you see me and I appear calm and serene, I may not really feel like that on the inside. But I know that composure works best for the staff and doctors and patients around me. That's who I am. I'll let you in on a little secret. Being a professional administrator requires a fair measure of professional *acting*. But perhaps you already knew that. I clearly see how you do the same kind of professional acting when puzzling over clinical problem you haven't solved yet. Or, when you are with a patient who is driving you a bit crazy.

Thanks for being on the same stage with me. It helps more than you know. More than we administrators like to admit.

Sincerely,
Your Administrator

Afterword

I was thrilled when Corinne and John asked me to write the epilogue for their new workbook, recognizing the tremendous expertise, complementary skill sets, and decades of management services and practice management consultation Corinne and John have brought, both independently and now in close collaboration, to the field of ophthalmology.

Corinne and John have spent the bulk of their remarkably successful careers doing fundamentally different things within the field of ophthalmology. Corinne having worked as a hospital administrator, and later as an ophthalmic practice administrator, and John in long-time service to the profession as a leading practice management consultant and resident "ophthalmologistologist." From these parallel career tracks, they have synthesized a new approach to practice excellence in this book. Their work underscores a truth about the practice of eye care that has always been hiding in plain sight: Even the most talented and productive ophthalmologists depend daily on the competency and performance of their managers and supervisors.

Even the most gifted ophthalmologists are not stand-alone all stars. They must be buttressed and supported by effective managers and supervisors. In this workbook, Corinne and John provide a tremendous value to our community, whether your role in that community is as a surgeon and practice owner, an administrator, a department head, or even a consultant to the profession.

Wohl C, Pinto JB. *UP: Taking Ophthalmic Administrators and Their Management Teams to the Next Level of Skill, Performance, and Career Satisfaction, Second Edition* (pp 291-292).

The authors have left few stones unturned. *UP* offers salient content regarding many complex, high-priority issues that administrators and managers face each day, and it will be especially helpful as a resource guide for the handling of more challenging situations, when, as I've heard John say, "You're drinking from a firehose with your hair on fire."

Don't think of this book as one-and-done reading. Don't just gather up a few high-level pearls and consign the book to your office shelf. I recommend that you keep this new book on your desk; refer to it frequently; make full use of the exercises and worksheets; recommend it to your staff, colleagues, and peers; and challenge yourself to keep striding down your career path. I know of no other workbook in our small corner of health care that is so comprehensive, sophisticated, and practical as *UP*. Everyone taking this workbook to heart and making full use of its content and development materials will progress in their management skills, effectiveness, productivity, and career satisfaction.

UP is derived from the 75 years of complementary professional experiences that Corinne and John have melded together here to shorten the learning curve of career-minded business professionals in ophthalmology. I commend it to you and wish you great success as you keep working and moving *UP*!

—Craig N. Piso, PhD
Wilkes-Barre, Pennsylvania

Craig N. Piso, PhD is the founder and president of Piso and Associates, LLC, an organizational development consulting firm based in Northeastern Pennsylvania. Dr. Piso is a Pennsylvania-licensed psychologist with training and experience since 1979 that has included family systems clinical practice, corporate managed behavioral health, and consultation within health care, business, and education. He is an author, contributing to numerous books and periodicals, and he is an award-winning presenter at diverse professional development conferences. Craig can be reached at (570) 239-3114 or cpiso@pisoandassociates.com.

Financial Disclosures

Suzanne D. Bruno has no financial or proprietary interest in the materials presented herein.

John B. Pinto is an ophthalmology practice management consultant in his firm, John Pinto & Associates, Inc.

Dr. Craig N. Piso has no financial or proprietary interest in the materials presented herein.

Corinne Wohl is an ophthalmology practice management consultant in her firm, C. Wohl & Associates, Inc.

Index

Made in the USA
Monee, IL
13 September 2026

62976962R00177